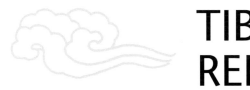

TIBETAN
RELAXATION

KUM NYE MASSAGE AND MOVEMENT

TARTHANG TULKU

TIBETAN RELAXATION

KUM NYE MASSAGE AND MOVEMENT

DUNCAN BAIRD PUBLISHERS

LONDON

Tibetan Relaxation
Tarthang Tulku

First published in the United Kingdom and Ireland in 2003 by
Duncan Baird Publishers Ltd
Sixth Floor
Castle House
75–76 Wells Street
London W1T 3QH

Material from this book was first published in the United States in 1978
by Dharma Publishing in two volumes illustrated with figure drawings:
Kum Nye Relaxation Part 1 (Theory, Preparation, Massage) and
Kum Nye Relaxation Part 2 (Movement Exercises).

The article "Kum Nye in Context: Buddhism and Tibetan Medicine", pp.14–15,
was prepared from materials submitted by the editors of Dharma Publishing.

Managing Editor: Judy Barratt
Editor: Lucy Latchmore
Designer: Dan Sturges
Picture Research: Cecilia Weston-Baker
Commissioned photography: Matthew Ward
Decorative Borders: Sally Taylor (artistpartners ltd)

British Library Cataloguing-in-Publication Data:
A CIP record for this book is available from the British Library.

ISBN: 1-904292-17-8

10 9 8 7 6 5 4 3 2

Typeset in Perpetua
Colour reproduction by Color & Print Gallery Sdn Bhd, Malaysia
Printed by Imago, Singapore

NOTES
Before following any advice or practice suggested in this book, it is
recommended that you consult your doctor as to its suitability, especially if
you are pregnant, or suffer from any health problems or special conditions.
The publishers, the author and the photographers cannot accept any
responsibility for any injuries or damage incurred as a result of following
the exercises in this book, or of using any of the therapeutic techniques
described or mentioned here. Essential oils must be diluted in a base oil
before use. They should not be taken internally and are for adult use only.

The abbreviations CE and BCE are used throughout this book:
CE Common Era (the equivalent of AD);
BCE Before the Common Era (the equivalent of BC).

Dedicated to everyone seeking harmony and balance –
the foundation for peace within, compassion for self and others,
and the activation of our potential for enlightenment.

May all beings be forever joined with happiness and the causes of happiness,

May all beings be forever free from suffering and the causes of suffering,

May all beings never be separated from the bliss that is free of suffering,

Freed from the confusions of dualistic mind, released from bondage to hatred and desire,

May all beings dwell in the quiet joy of equanimity.

TRADITIONAL BUDDHIST PRAYER

CONTENTS

INTRODUCTION

"When we learn to open our senses and touch our feelings directly, our bodies and minds make full contact with one another, and all our experiences become richer, healthier and more fulfilling."

Kum Nye (pronounced Koom Nyay) comprises a series of simple but effective healing exercises that work to relieve stress, transform negative behavioural patterns, promote balance and health, and increase our enjoyment and appreciation of life. The exercises are based on theories of the gross and subtle energy systems of the body, which underpin Tibetan medicine and the body–mind disciplines of Buddhism.

In modern times, confusion, chaos and overstimulation have become such a feature of daily activity that we are often too tense and charged up to enjoy life. Kum Nye works to counter this effect: opening our senses and our hearts so that we feel satisfied and fulfilled, able to appreciate every aspect of our lives more fully. By practising Kum Nye, we can enrich the quality of our experience as we learn to live more harmoniously.

As a young boy, I grew up in the Nyingma tradition (*nyingma*, meaning "ancient ones", is the oldest of the four Tibetan Buddhist traditions) in eastern Tibet. My father was a physician and a lama, and it was he who first introduced me to Kum Nye. However, Kum Nye was not well known in Tibet and was most often practised as an adjunct to other practices. My gurus sometimes taught the basic theory and practice of Kum Nye as a preparatory practice for meditation. However, until now Kum Nye has had no systematized body of written instructions and, consequently, my practice of Kum Nye has always had a distinct flavour of exploration and experimentation.

The unique value of the Kum Nye system of relaxation is that it views the body and mind holistically, working to integrate and balance the physical and the psychological to achieve health. Kum Nye achieves this by relaxing and healing our bodies and minds, bringing their energies together to function calmly and smoothly. Because it leads to the integration of body and mind in all activities, the relaxation of Kum Nye is more vital and lasting than the feeling of well-being experienced during ordinary physical exercise: when we learn to open our senses and touch our feelings directly, our bodies and minds make full contact with one another, and all our experiences become richer, healthier and more fulfilling. As we become more deeply acquainted with ourselves, growing in self-understanding, we are also able to share more fully with others.

Although a predominantly oral tradition, the practices of Kum Nye are referred to in Tibetan medical texts as ways of healing diseases that result from energy blockages. Kum Nye is also described in general terms in the *Vinaya* texts of Buddhism (originating in India, these teachings guided the conduct of monks and nuns), which suggest ways to relieve the fatigue experienced during long periods of meditation. Kum Nye is thus part of the lineage of medical and spiritual theories and practices that links Tibetan with Indian and Chinese medicine. This lineage has given rise to many disciplines, such as yoga and acupuncture, and forms the roots of many of the more recent body–mind disciplines.

Although based on original Kum Nye principles, the Kum Nye Relaxation system presented in this book is thoroughly modern, drawn from my own experience and adapted specifically to suit modern needs. I have used the open aspect of Kum Nye to make adaptations based on the knowledge and understanding gained during my broad education at a number of major monasteries in both eastern and central Tibet. (This education included study of Tibetan medicine, as well as strictly Buddhist treatises.) These adaptations have culminated in the complete system of exercises that I call "Kum Nye Relaxation" (a name used to distinguish the system from the original Kum Nye practices).

The impulse to develop Kum Nye Relaxation came when I moved to California, USA, in 1969. Arriving in Berkeley, I began holding ceremonies and offering classes. Within a few months I founded the Tibetan Nyingma Meditation Center, which offered classes in essential Buddhist teachings, Tibetan language and philosophy. In 1972, as interest in Tibetan teachings grew, I founded the Nyingma Institute. There I offered an eight-week intensive summer session known as the Human Development Training Retreat.

Fully prepared to introduce traditional meditation techniques, I was surprised to discover that many of the participants experienced difficulties with extended periods of sitting because of restlessness, mental distractions and various kinds of physical discomfort. To help them overcome these difficulties, I introduced them to some of the Kum Nye massage and movement exercises that I had learned in Tibet. The results of these experiments were obviously beneficial: participants who had unsuccessfully attempted to meditate for months, or even years, were able to quiet body and mind using these exercises.

Since then I have developed several hundred exercises that my Western students have found particularly helpful. Many of the exercises had to be adapted to suit the specific needs and problems faced by Westerners. However, over the course of the years, with students practising the various exercises, writing about their experiences and discussing them in class, certain exercises emerged as being particularly beneficial. This book includes the simplest and most effective of these exercises, all of which can be practised safely by anyone, young or old, without a teacher. Sitting, breathing, self-massage and different kinds of movement exercises are included.

I hope that this book will introduce the benefits of Kum Nye to many people of various backgrounds and interests, and will assist them in developing and continuing their experience of inner relaxation. I also hope that delight in the discovery of many as yet undeveloped aspects of Kum Nye will enrich the practice of Western students and eventually encourage systematization in Western terms. Finally, this book is intended as a practical guide to the deep pleasure of a healthy and balanced life, rich in beauty and enjoyment, and leading to harmony for all beings, even in these difficult times.

HOW TO USE THIS BOOK

"Adopt a spirit of openness at all times: simply do the exercise, reflect on the experience, do it again. Relax, repeat this process and understanding will come."

This book is intended as a beginner's guide to Kum Nye Relaxation. The structure of the book is designed to help you navigate your way through the wide range of exercises and build a practice that is tailored to your specific needs, problems and disposition. The book is divided into six chapters. In the first chapter we are introduced to the practice of Kum Nye. We discover the context of Kum Nye: its roots in the Buddhist traditions of India; its development in Tibet; and its basis in the Ayurvedic and Tibetan medical traditions. In particular we examine the Tibetan concept of the body on which the healing of Kum Nye is predicated. Next we explore the essential principles of Kum Nye and its relevance in the modern world, before looking at the nature of the practice itself, the different types of exercises it involves and their various stages of progression. Finally we prepare ourselves for starting a practice, examining the ideal practice environment, and the equipment and clothing that are needed, as well as our mental attitudes and guidelines for establishing a practice.

Chapter two is concerned with the sitting and breathing exercises, which constitute the cornerstone of Kum Nye. They provide a starting point for practice: the sitting exercises introduce us to the attitudes of awareness, concentration and openness that are central to the practice; the breathing exercises help us to develop the specific Kum Nye breathing technique, which should be performed during all the other exercises and ultimately throughout daily life. These exercises also represent the culmination of Kum Nye, for when performed properly they offer a starting point for meditation, the practice for which Kum Nye is a preparation.

The third chapter presents a wide range of massages, each one dedicated to a particular part of the body. In addition to general massages, there are also more detailed massages geared toward specific acupressure points. To help you locate these points, maps of the relevant body parts are supplied, with the points marked by numbered dots.

Chapter four provides a starting point for movement practice. It introduces some of the simplest of the movement exercises from which the beginner can develop a basic movement practice. Once you have established your foundation practice in chapter four, chapters five and six offer you a chance to gradually broaden and extend your repertoire of exercises, with a selection of different exercises ranging from the simple to the more advanced.

To enable you to tailor your practice to your level of experience and ability, all the movement exercises are graded according to level of difficulty – level one exercises being the easiest, and level three the most advanced. The level of a particular exercise is indicated by a circular motif (see key, opposite) located above the exercise heading. Chapter four includes level one and two exercises, whereas chapters five and six include exercises at all three levels of difficulty. All the exercises at a particular level are equivalent in terms of difficulty, regardless of the chapter, allowing you to mix and match exercises from different chapters if you choose.

Some of the movement exercises offer special features designed to help you gain more from your practice. Blue boxes present variations of the main exercise, offering opportunities for developing the exercise further. Peach-coloured boxes provide complementary instructions to those in the main exercise, encouraging you to deepen your experience by expanding your feelings and sensations. Tips marked out in bold offer more practical advice, with remedies and solutions to problems and difficulties commonly experienced during certain exercises.

The organization of the book, as it is explained here, allows us to develop our practice at our own pace. The clear structure offers guidance to beginners as they establish a practice, as well as a level of flexibility that allows more advanced students to develop their relaxation practice as they choose.

As a beginner the simplest way to structure your practice is to follow the guidelines on p.25. These suggest starting with a couple of sitting and breathing exercises, a massage and a selection of the simplest movement exercises from chapter four. From there you can develop your practice at your own pace, broadening your repertoire of exercises gradually, attempting more difficult, level three exercises when you feel ready.

As well as offering variety to those who are easily bored, this broad-based approach is ideal for those who find it difficult to perform the sitting and breathing exercises. The massage and movement exercises ease the physical discomfort that makes sitting still impossible, and they develop the mental concentration required for the meditative aspects of the sitting and breathing exercises.

Once you are familiar with the various exercises, you are free to structure your practice as you wish, opting for whatever strategy suits your state of being on a particular day. For example, if you have spent the day rushing from one activity to the next, it can be refreshing to devote most of your practice time to simply sitting and breathing, observing whatever is happening inside. On the other hand, if you are extremely agitated, you may find it easiest to begin your practice with some self-massage, before attempting any of the more focused exercises.

Feel free to move back and forth between the chapters, allowing the wisdom of your body to dictate the exercises that you practise on a particular day. Sometimes you may wish to work more generally on the different parts of your body, perhaps with self-massages for the head and face, combined with a movement exercise involving the torso and arms, and another involving the lower body. Alternatively, you could work on one specific body part: for example, with a massage for the hips, followed by an exercise that focuses on that area of the body.

In a class setting the teacher may suggest an order of practice that is especially effective in stimulating complementary energies, but you can trust your own impulses. Kum Nye is an open exploration, not a prescriptive healing art. There is a tendency in the West to expect teachers to provide us with all the answers, to reveal objective truths about the nature of our experiences: what they should be; how they should feel; what benefits they should bring us. However, the approach in Kum Nye, as it is in many Eastern traditions, is quite the reverse: a teacher does not express certain kinds of knowledge until the student reaches a point of understanding for himself or herself. Then the teacher confirms that this is so. Everybody's experience is unique, and everybody has the capacity to find their way to truth. For this reason it is important to enter each exercise without expectations, for these can limit your experience of the exercise. Adopt a spirit of openness at all times: simply do the exercise, reflect on the experience, do it again. Relax, repeat this process and understanding will come.

SYMBOLS USED IN THIS BOOK

Level one exercises (beginner)

Level two exercises (intermediate)

Level three exercises (advanced)

▶   Exercise continued overleaf

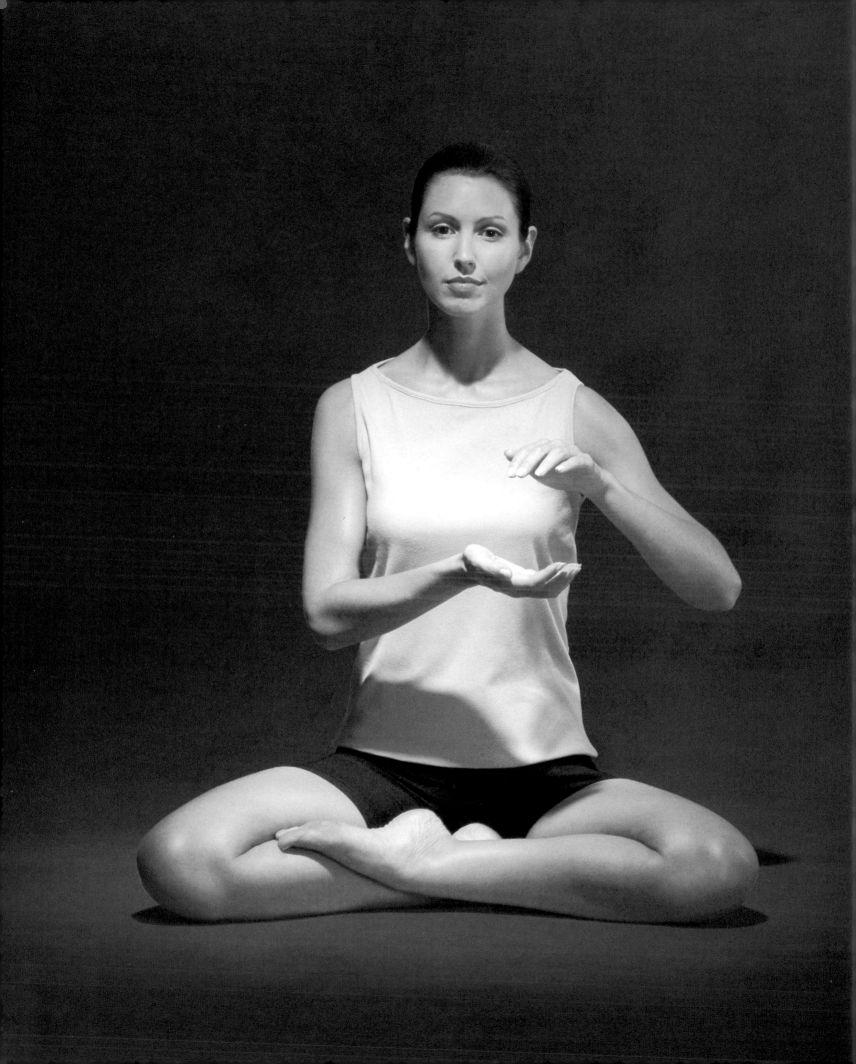

CHAPTER ONE

DISCOVERING KUM NYE

*"Through relaxation we develop a whole
new way of being."*

Kum Nye is an ancient Tibetan healing system that aims to harmonize and integrate mind and body, self and world. This is achieved by stimulating, releasing and expanding the subtle energies of feeling that unite the mind, body and senses. In this chapter we begin by tracing the history and context of Kum Nye, examining its origins, development and relationship to other Tibetan traditions. Next we learn the basic principles of Kum Nye, gaining an understanding of its place in modern life. We explore the practice of Kum Nye in detail, finding out about the various types of exercise and the stages of progression that these involve. We finish with practical preparation for our practice, paying attention to our surroundings, our mental attitudes and the structure and development of our practice.

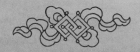

KUM NYE IN CONTEXT: BUDDHISM AND TIBETAN MEDICINE

"Healing the body by integrating and balancing the physical, mental and emotional aspects of our embodiment is an important step toward the more profound healing of enlightenment in which wholeness is restored to human consciousness."

The system of Kum Nye Relaxation presented in this book is grounded in a system of healing transmitted for nearly twelve hundred years within the Buddhist culture of Tibet. We can trace the link between healing and Buddhism to the time of the Buddha, who lived in India during the sixth to fifth centuries BCE. The Buddha (literally meaning "The Awakened One") is renowned for attaining the state of complete, perfect enlightenment while meditating at the foot of the Bodhi Tree at Bodh Gaya, in India. From this realization came teachings that were disseminated over the course of forty-five years. Passed on since then by unbroken lineages of masters for over 2,500 years, these teachings form the heart of all Buddhist traditions.

The central purpose of Buddhism is to gain freedom from the suffering that afflicts humanity: suffering of isolation, fragmentation and separation from others based on an incorrect notion of self; and suffering of change in the face of the impermanence of all existence. Freedom comes from recognizing the true nature of our being, expanding the scope of our knowledge beyond the material and physical realms, and understanding our interconnection with all modes of existence. In this context, healing the body by integrating and balancing the physical, mental and emotional aspects of our embodiment can be understood as an important step toward the more profound healing of enlightenment in which wholeness (in the widest universal sense) is restored to human consciousness.

From Ayurveda to Tibetan medicine

Ayurveda, the traditional medical system of Ancient India, is the principal healing system associated with Buddhism. Ayurvedic medical practices were first alluded to in the *Vedas* (sacred Hindu texts) and initially comprised a disparate array of herbal remedies and incantations. However, between the sixth century BCE and the eighth century CE, Ayurveda developed into a systematized body of medical knowledge. This was achieved largely as a result of the increasingly sophisticated meditation techniques that developed during this period, which sharpened powers of introspection, revealing insights into the workings of the body on a subtle energetic level.

Both Buddhism and Ayurveda were introduced into Tibet during the seventh century by a great Tibetan king, called Songtsen Gampo. After Songtsen unified the tribes of Tibet, he devoted himself to developing Tibetan culture by drawing on the wisdom and traditions of the great civilizations surrounding Tibet, including Persia, India, China and Nepal. At that time Tibet had no written language so the King sent one of his ministers, Thon-mi Sambhota, to India to learn Sanskrit and develop a system of writing. Thon-mi accomplished his mission, returning to Tibet with a language system and Buddhist texts that he and the King worked together to translate.

In the eighth century a second king – Trisong Detsen – worked to bring Buddhism to his people, inviting India's greatest masters to Tibet and sending Tibetans to India for training. Over the course of a few generations, nearly a thousand Sanskrit texts were translated into Tibetan. As well as the original words of the Buddha, these texts included the commentaries and treatises of the great Buddhist masters, which featured systems of philosophy, logic and grammar, governance, the ritual arts and sciences, as well as Ayurvedic medicine. Since then these teachings have gradually been assimilated into Tibetan culture. The original theories of Ayurvedic medicine, combined with other influences, were adapted, developed and shaped into the distinct system of Tibetan medicine practised today.

The concepts of Tibetan medicine

Tibetan medicine, like Ayurveda, is based on the concept that health depends on a delicate balance of vital life forces. In Tibetan medicine these are known as the three humours – equivalent to the *doshas* of the Ayurvedic system from which they developed. The three humours – wind, bile and phlegm – are principles of life energy that govern all the processes of the body, physiological, mental and emotional. They encompass both the constituents of the physical body and the energy networks of the subtle body. For example, wind has the qualities of motion, lightness and dryness and predominates in the abdomen and lower body. It governs movement, respiration, digestion, reproduction and thought, and affects vitality, mental clarity and gynecological function.

The subtle body comprises a network of more than 72,000 energy channels. The most important channel is the central *dhuma* or "vein", which runs from the top of the head down the length of the spinal column. Running either side of the *dhuma* are the *ro-ma* and the *rkyang-ma*. (These three channels correspond respectively to the *sushumna*, the *ida* and the *pingala nadis* in Ayurvedic medicine.) The side channels spiral around the *dhuma*, intersecting at six key points called *chakras*. These are the main energy centres of the body, responsible for distributing energy throughout the subtle anatomy. They are located on the crown of the head; in the centre of the brow; at the base of the throat; in the centre of the chest near the heart; by the navel; and by the genitals. These positions coincide with important nerve plexuses (networks) along the spinal cord.

Kum Nye and Tibetan medicine

When all three humours are in balance, energy flows freely through the *chakras* and channels of the subtle body, the physical body is strong and healthy, the mind calm and clear, the emotions stable. However, negative thoughts, harmful actions, improper behaviour and inappropriate diet are believed to cause humoral imbalances and energy blockages, resulting in physical diseases and mental and emotional problems.

In Tibet, Kum Nye was developed alongside other medical practices as a way of healing the body, using breathing techniques, self-massages, specific postures and movement exercises to rebalance the humours and release energy blockages at all levels of embodiment. Because of its ability to ease the physical body and calm the mind and emotions, Kum Nye was also utilized by Buddhist practitioners as a preliminary to meditation and other advanced yogic practices.

This rug depicts the Myrobalan Tree (also known as the Medicine Tree or Tree of Life), which is the King of Medicines in Ayurvedic traditions. According to 8th-century Tibetan writings, the tree's roots, stem, branches, bark, leaves and fruit formed the basis of medical compounds used to treat disease.

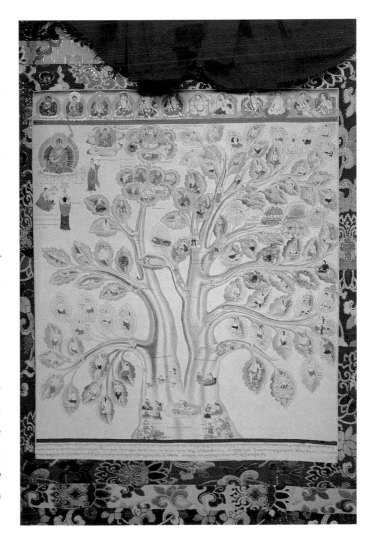

THE BALANCE OF KUM NYE

*"Kum Nye is the art of developing balance by
integrating body, mind, senses and environment."*

We all have memories of times when we have felt particularly alive, when the world has seemed fresh and promising, like a garden on a bright spring morning. Whatever the circumstances leading to such moments, there is often a sense of acute vitality, supported by an awareness that all elements are in absolute harmony: the air seems to pulse with life; our bodies feel healthy and energetic; our minds are clear and confident. There is a lucent quality to our perception and every feature of the environment pleases our senses: colours appear especially vivid, sounds are melodious and odours fragrant. All aspects of our experience seem to blend perfectly as we relax, allowing the boundaries between inner and outer space to become fluid. Nothing is fixed and we feel spacious and open, acting with perfect ease and appropriateness.

The essence of this experience is balance and its offshoot is a deep feeling of nurturance, refreshment and wholeness that extends far beyond the feeling that we ordinarily call happiness. Kum Nye is the art of developing this balance by integrating body, mind, senses and environment. This is achieved through a gentle yet profound process of relaxation involving the release of physical, mental and emotional tensions and blockages in order to cultivate the free flow of feeling and sensation throughout the body. By consciously focusing on and expanding these energies both within and beyond ourselves, we move closer to their source – the vitality of the universe itself. In so doing we discover a whole new way of being, an open perspective that enables us to appreciate the wholesome quality of complete, lived experience.

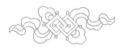

The loss of balance in the modern world

When we are open to the beauty of the world, it seems natural to live in mutual harmony and union with the universe. As young children many of us will have experienced such harmony, but as we grow we are encouraged to foster our personalities too intensely, deepening feelings of separation and individuality at the expense of the warmth and security of communality and connection that our hearts desire. The pressures and complications of modern society render it difficult to do otherwise: to be successful in business, in friendship, even in play, we are often forced into competitive and stressful situations that promote feelings of alienation and anxiety.

This separation occurs not only between self and world, but also between body and mind: not realizing the importance of integrating both body and mind in all our activities, we emphasize either intellectual achievement or the physical form of the body at the expense of the rich feelings and sensations that link the two.

When we restrict our feelings and sensations in this way, we prevent these energies from giving us the sustenance we need to be healthy and happy. Instead we seek satisfaction outside ourselves. We may be drawn to exciting activities that stimulate our minds and senses, but leave us wanting more. We may seek solace in drugs, such as alcohol or hallucinogens, or even turn to the spiritual path, hoping at last to be truly nurtured, only to discover that here, too, we remain dissatisfied. In this way we waste our energies, jumping from experience to experience, from thought to thought, constantly reliving the past or planning for the future. Lost in daydreams, we catch glimpses of pleasure or rich sensation, but full contact always eludes us.

We may attempt to regain a sense of wholeness through ownership of our families, property or material wealth, in this way trying to exert control over our lives. However, such control is artificial and out of touch with the natural laws and cycles that govern our bodies, minds and the world around us. It leaves us feeling trapped and unfulfilled, alienated from that with which we seek connection – ourselves, our loved ones, the universe itself.

Kum Nye and the rediscovery of balance

A sense of unfulfilment arises when we cut ourselves off from the full experience of ourselves and our world. Through neglect our senses toughen like elephant's hide, diminishing the fullness of our sensory capacity. Only when we soften this toughness by developing the energies of feeling and sensation that link body to mind, self to world, do we open to the full field of experience - the source of satisfaction.

The exercises of Kum Nye work to soften us in this way, bringing us into harmony with ourselves and the world around us. When we reach this state of balance we are able to participate in the natural flow of the universe: we come to understand that we depend on nature, and nature – indeed the whole universe – depends on us. Like all other living organisms in the universe, we form complete units or systems composed of smaller interrelated units, such as the skeletal, muscular and nervous systems. These in turn comprise yet smaller units, which can be subdivided right down to the subtlest energetic level. From the subatomic to the cosmic, the smooth functioning of each system relies on the functioning of the others: all are intimately connected, created alike from the same basic energies that comprise the universe.

When we acknowledge these interrelationships, we recognize the importance of creating harmony both within and without ourselves. We realize that we possess the resources needed to find both balance and happiness, for our bodies and minds serve as channels for the vital energies of the cosmos. By slowing down and relaxing through the exercises of Kum Nye, we

Prayer wheels contain written mantras – syllables that subliminally transmit the energy of the awakened mind, promoting balance and harmony among living beings as well as natural forces. Activated by the motion of prayer wheels, these mantras calm the mind and open the heart, calling forth deep feelings that restore us spiritually and simulate our vital energies.

learn to develop these resources: opening our bodies and minds to the experience of feeling and sensation. As we work to expand these energies, we discover the naturally alert and fluid state of the body and mind, and find our connection to the world around us. With our body, mind and senses integrated, all our actions, ideas and movements become flowing and harmonious. We develop greater awareness, which gives us the freedom to take charge of our lives – not in a forceful or grasping way, but with rightful confidence. Increasingly sensitive to those around us, we naturally do what is appropriate and beneficial. We seek to function in a positive way in the world, aware that ideas and actions that result in stability and happiness for ourselves contribute also to the balance and harmony of the world around us.

THE PRACTICE OF KUM NYE

*"Kum Nye practices are symbols that point us
to the nature of all existence."*

The word "Kum" means body or embodiment. "Nye" means massage or interaction. In Tibetan, *lu* refers to our physical body; *ku*, to a higher, more subtle body. When we practise Kum Nye, we activate the *ku* by stimulating feeling in the *lu*, or physical body. This cultivation of feeling is the massage or interaction of Nye.

Usually when we speak of "massage" we mean the physical action of pressing, rubbing and manipulating the body. In Kum Nye the word is used more generally to refer to the process by which subtle feeling-tones or energies are released so that they flow freely throughout the body, integrating the mental and the physical, relating feeling to form. These energies behave like a moving, vibrating aura, which runs through us, outward from us and surrounds us. We discover true relaxation as we learn to heal ourselves with these energies, releasing tensions and blockages, harmonizing all aspects of our being.

The exercises of Kum Nye

In Kum Nye, there are various ways, involving both stillness and movement, to stimulate the flow of feeling and sensation that leads to true relaxation. We begin by developing stillness of body, breath and mind (see chapter two). Simply sitting still and relaxing gives us a chance to appreciate feelings of which we are normally unaware. This relaxation is then subtly aided by breathing simultaneously through the nose and mouth so gently and evenly that we are hardly conscious of inhaling and exhaling at all – a breathing technique that allows us to contact the positive vitality of the throat centre (see p.31).

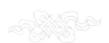

To encourage the breath to become calm, rhythmic and quiet, we focus our awareness on the body, with the result that distracting thoughts and images are banished from the mind and the whole body comes alive. It is at this point that we first become aware of our bodies on a subtle energetic level as we focus on the feelings and sensations that pervade our bodies.

Once aware of these subtle energies, we can draw on self-massage techniques (see chapter three) and a wide selection of movement exercises (see chapters four to six) to develop the process of relaxation further. Pressing and rubbing certain points on the body, moving slowly in certain ways, or producing and releasing tension in particular postures, enables us to stimulate the flow of these physical energies, releasing areas of tension caused by energy blockages. As our contact with our feelings and sensations increases, we can in turn use these energies to contact deeper, yet more subtle energies on a mental, emotional and ultimately spiritual level. The deeper and richer our experience of this self-generating energy massage becomes, the more it occurs naturally throughout our daily lives. Gradually we discover a calm, clear, deepening quality of all-pervading energy that vitalizes every sense, feeling, thought and activity, enabling us to feel directly the interconnections between breath, senses, body and mind. This is the feeling to expand and accumulate – the essence of Kum Nye.

The stages of relaxation

There are three levels at which each Kum Nye exercise may be experienced, corresponding to three different levels of relaxation. At the first level feelings possess an obvious physical or emotional tone such as warmth or coolness, joy or sadness.

These feelings are easy to identify and describe: there may be a tingling sensation, a slightly painful sensation or perhaps a feeling of relaxation and energy flowing through the body. These are surface feelings. We feel them in particular locations in the body, and we remain aware of the self experiencing these feelings during the exercise.

By paying close attention to these initial feelings or sensations, we can use them to penetrate to a deeper level of feeling where we are able to detect blocks in the flow of energy. Such blockages cannot be identified in emotional or physical terms, rather they are characterized by a holding quality, a sense of density and toughness. While this layer of feeling is more difficult to deepen than the first, the blockages can be gently melted through a kind of open concentration. At this stage,

there is a sense of the exercise doing itself, although there continues to be an awareness of the self feeling the sensations. However, this self may be experienced as less solid.

As we contact the third level of feeling, we broach the realm of pure energy or experience, where all residues of patterning are transcended. At this stage there are no longer any feelings that can be separated out and identified, only a fluid, melting quality akin to the boundlessness of overwhelming joy. This quality is without time or place: we do not know what it is, where it is, or how it is happening, for at this level the

When the energies of body and mind converge, they illuminate the inner landscapes of human experience, dispelling tension, awakening joy, inspiring vision and empowering thought and action.

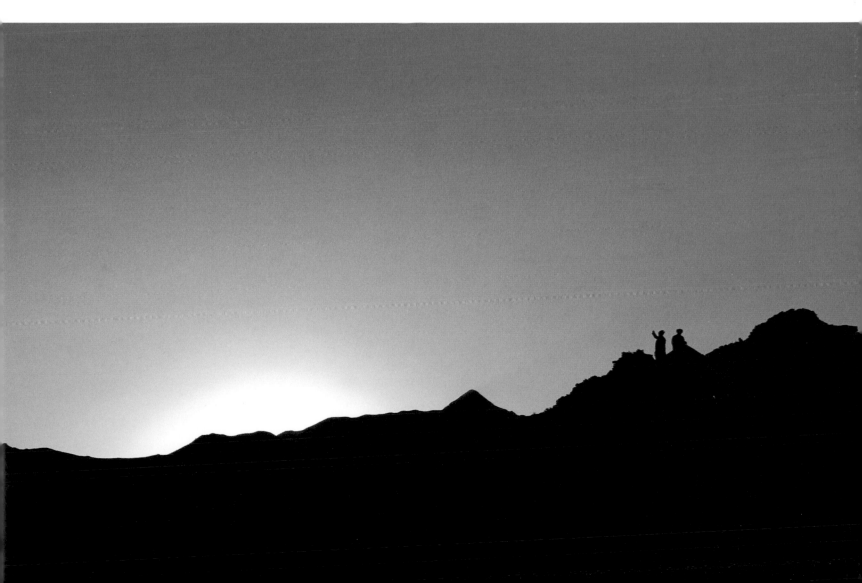

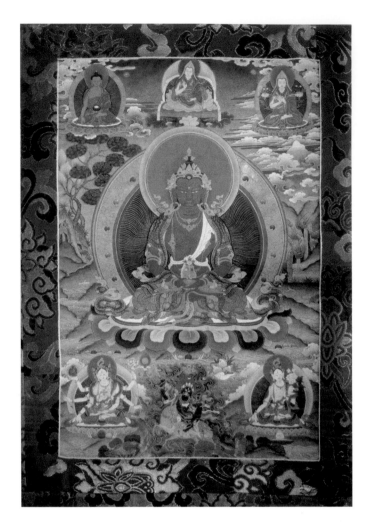

Amitayus is the Buddha of Infinite Life and embodies supreme healing power. His body is a deep red, signifying profound compassion, and he holds a jar filled with the elixir of immortality. Amitayus belongs to the Longevity Trinity, which protects against spiritual ills and prolongs life, increasing opportunities for benevolent action and the attainment of enlightenment.

individual ego no longer exists; we have become the feeling, totally at one with it. This is the stage of fruition, the point of completion that is true relaxation.

The opening of the senses

Central to this process of relaxation is the opening up of the senses to new channels and dimensions of sensation. When this occurs, every part of the body becomes vibrantly alive. We discover that it is possible to experience ecstatic beauty at every moment of our lives, as if we were forever hearing beautiful music or gazing upon the finest works of art.

Our habitual way of perceiving the world is transformed. When seeing, we move beyond surfaces, concentrating our awareness lightly on the objects that surround us so that we sense feelings from their forms. By broadening our gaze in this way, we invite an ecstatic interaction between the subtle inner energies of our bodies and the outer energies of the objects that surround us. With this our perceptions of a separate subject and object, a "seer" and a seen, break down. Instead there is only vision, the ongoing process of seeing that is a constant expression of a vital totality.

In a similar way we learn to contact and appreciate sound so that we sense the vibrations as they penetrate our bodies, using them to stimulate harmonious interactions between ourselves and the surrounding universe. Listening to soft music, we allow the gentle vibrations to relax and soothe us, releasing energies that can heal us at deeper levels of our consciousness. When speaking, all our sounds are gentle so that there can be no shocking or destructive quality to our communication.

Eating becomes a true meeting of the senses with their object – a ceremonial act of appreciation in which we enjoy the different feeling-tones of tastes, smells, textures and colours, distributing them throughout the body and beyond.

The sweetness bred by fully exercising our senses in this way can be expanded more and more each day. Without any fixed goal, almost without conscious effort, we open our senses to the full breadth and beauty of sensual experience, allowing our bodies to surrender to the joyful sensation that this brings. The quality of this feeling is mild and sweet like milk and honey; it touches us deeply, expanding within us until we enjoy an almost overwhelming feeling of fulfilment. As these feelings and sensations expand in space and time, they activate energy that massages the outside as well as inside of our bodies, integrating inner and outer aspects of our being, attuning us to all aspects of our surroundings and promoting a deep inner peace.

The power to transform energy

Once we tap into the deepest levels of relaxation, we come to view all sensations and emotions with a playful, open attitude. We realize that beneath every feeling or sensation, whether negative or positive, happy or sad, there lies the same pure energy. With this knowledge comes the power to transform surface energies from one form into another, from the negative to the positive, the sad to the happy. It is a power that enables us to heal our grasping, shadow side, the unbalanced part of the psyche that springs from an underlying sense of inadequacy. We can recognize that part of ourselves whenever we become trapped in damaging patterns of behaviour, thought or emotion, whenever we are plagued with recurrent feelings of insecurity, worthlessness and failure. We can transform these negative feelings into a positive sense of abundance and fulfilment by embracing them, accepting them as simple manifestations of energy and so penetrating through their negative quality to the neutrality of pure energy beyond.

Once assimilated, the techniques of Kum Nye can positively transform the way that we process our everyday experiences. At the beginning of any sensation, whether negative or positive, we increase and expand it until it becomes firmly established. When we reach the second layer of feeling we expand that as well, experiencing it fully until we pass into the final stage. When the next feeling or sensation arises, we begin once again, creating a continuously cycling energy massage. In this way energy constantly refreshes itself and the patterns of existence – the patterns of our living being – are constantly renewed. Neither time nor age can catch and freeze this energy, for it is forever moving and refreshing itself, never delayed or at a standstill.

When we really know how to quicken and develop the subtle energies of feelings and sensations, cultivating their potential so that they continuously feed and nourish themselves in an ever-expanding, flowing way, it is even possible to refine, recreate and regenerate all of the patterns of the living organism, ensuring a long, healthy and fulfilling life. By increasing our awareness of the immediate feeling-tone of each sensation, Kum Nye teaches us to move within these forms of energy so that we become familiar with different sensory levels, before finally contacting the neutral yet totally wholesome energy that pervades all forms.

Kum Nye and the nature of existence

The practice of Kum Nye serves as a methodology that awakens us to the nature of existence itself. By working with the energies within our bodies, we begin to understand how mind and matter function and interact. We develop an understanding of physical laws – how sensations arise, perceptions develop, concepts come into being and mental events take place. Once we become aware of the energy that pervades all existence, we are able to see, pursue and experience the potential of this energy. We appreciate the dynamic and vibrant character of the material world and draw upon this vitality to nourish ourselves.

Through feelings and sensations (the energy embodied in physical form) we learn to experience the physical patterns occurring in our bodies and from this understand how matter itself is patterned. We no longer see our bodies as fixed, solid things; instead we experience ourselves as an ongoing process of embodiment that at any given moment manifests itself as a physical entity and has the capability to continuously regenerate itself. As soon as we understand that the body is not a physical machine but rather an embodiment of values and responsiveness that takes part in a cosmic web of relations, we begin to understand and express a way of being that transcends the usual polarity between existence and non-existence.

Within this framework, energy is no longer seen as something that can be quantified and measured, something that adopts a specific form. Rather it is conceived as a limitless, seamless whole – an infinite force without beginning or end, inside or outside, pervading all, connecting all. Once we understand ourselves, we understand others; indeed we understand the nature of the universe, for the energies of our bodies are the energies of the universe.

PREPARING FOR PRACTICE

*"Even the moment practice begins, you are planting
the seed of a healthy, positive attitude."*

The practice of Kum Nye is an exploration and balancing of our inner environment. Our internal state of mind is reflected in our external environment so, before practising Kum Nye, it is important to make our external environment as harmonious as possible. This helps to encourage positive feelings during the practice. As our experience of our inner world expands through practice of Kum Nye, as we become more balanced, our appreciation of our external world increases effortlessly. With continuing practice, the separation between external and internal gradually melts away, and we naturally interact harmoniously with our environment.

Creating the right space and mood

Choose a clean, quiet place, either indoors or outdoors, where you will not be interrupted or distracted. The temperature should be comfortable, neither too hot nor too cold, and the lighting soft. A comfortable floor or a level grassy place make practice especially pleasant. If you are practising indoors, you may wish to open a window to clear the air, or burn some incense. Before you begin, take time to become familiar or reacquainted with your surroundings. Walk as well as look around, investigating any possible distractions until you feel comfortable about turning your attention inward.

For the sitting exercises you will need a cushion so that your pelvis is higher than your legs. If you find sitting on the ground too difficult, use a straight-backed chair instead. When performing the standing exercises, stand on a carpet or on the bare floor, not on a thick mat. For the self-massage, use a massage cream (lightly scented if you wish), or a vegetable oil such as safflower or olive. If you use vegetable oil, you may want to add a sweet scent, perhaps musk or cinnamon oil.

Before beginning your practice, remove anything that could obstruct movement or energy flow, such as your watch and any jewelry, spectacles or contact lenses. For the movement exercises wear a leotard or comfortable clothing that gives you maximum freedom of movement. For the self-massages either remove all of your clothes or wear loose-fitting garments that you can easily open to make contact with your skin.

Creating an environment that is conducive to practice is an expression of a positive attitude toward oneself. Intrinsic to practising Kum Nye exercises is the decision to find inner satisfaction. Nourish this attitude and it will grow within you, developing your sense of balance, happiness and relaxation.

Developing internal awareness

All the exercises in this book offer ways to touch and expand inner feelings and energies. The external form of the exercise may be stillness, breathing, self-massage or movement, but the internal exercise, the "energy massage" of Kum Nye, is concerned with the flow of feeling.

From the moment you begin your practice, focus on experiencing the feelings and sensations that arise rather than thinking analytically about what you are doing. Consider your posture and gestures as part of the quality of your experience and be aware of how they affect your feelings. When you move, do so slowly and rhythmically so that you can savour the joy of your discoveries. Execute each motion with gentle concentration – a kind of openness that encourages awareness.

Your experience will have an open-ended quality when you practise in this way, for as you perform an exercise, you will be aware of the form, texture and movement of the subtle feelings in your body. Feelings of dullness give way to an increased sensitivity to subtle muscular adjustments and energies; deep insights are then possible.

Participate in each exercise as fully as you can, involving your whole being – your heart, senses, awareness, feelings and

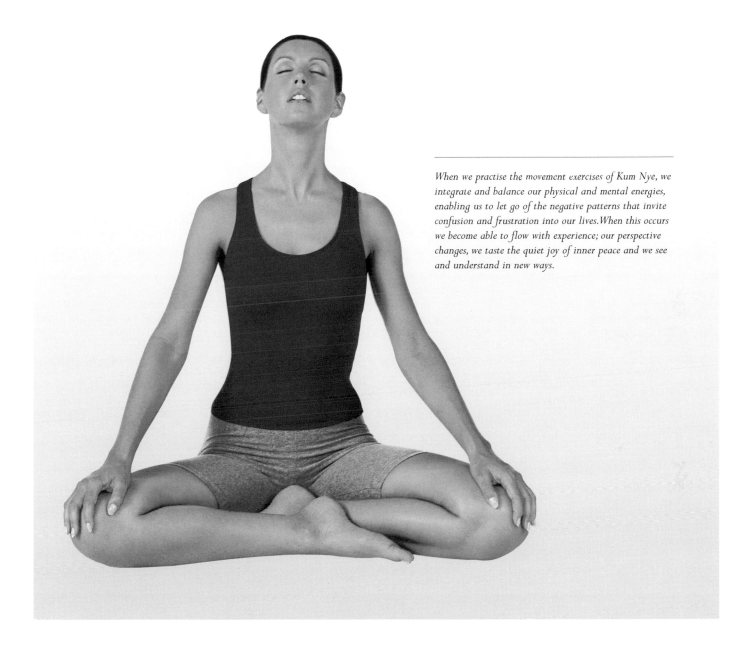

When we practise the movement exercises of Kum Nye, we integrate and balance our physical and mental energies, enabling us to let go of the negative patterns that invite confusion and frustration into our lives. When this occurs we become able to flow with experience; our perspective changes, we taste the quiet joy of inner peace and we see and understand in new ways.

consciousness. Bring all of yourself into the form of the exercise, allowing your negative as well as your positive feelings to be part of the experience. When you feel something, keep the energy of the feeling alive as long as possible, allowing it to expand and fill you. Broaden your feelings, letting them expand in every dimension of time and space.

The experience of each exercise has three characteristics: positive, negative and neutral. These terms are not judgments; it is as important to feel and work with negative qualities as it is to work with positive ones. Awareness of these qualities is an important part of each exercise: positive feeling can be recognized as a warm, soft and gentle sensation located primarily in the heart area; negative feeling tends to manifest itself as a dull, dark heaviness in the lower abdomen; neutral feeling possesses a quality of light, balanced stillness, which permeates the entire body and beyond into the surrounding space.

With time you will discover different levels of feeling and experience, until eventually you gain awareness of the energy that is present within every atom and molecule of your being. When this occurs you can increase your contact with this energy until every part of your body becomes a source of energy. Once you realize that energy is without location, that it is abundant and available at any time, you can truly experience the integration of body and mind.

Approach each exercise openly, without expectation or judgment, for if you begin an exercise with an expectation of a modality, you may cut yourself off from the experience. The key to practising Kum Nye is not to label, manipulate or try to make feelings mean something. When a judgment arises in your mind, use it as a signal to go deeper into sensations and feelings. Observe what organs, tissues and muscles are awakening; go into these places and explore. Do you feel pain, or joy, perhaps warmth or energy? What is the nature of the experience, the tones and the qualities?

Although this experience of full participation can be called mindfulness, consciousness or awareness, its nature is not concerned with naming and defining for there is no longer a critical mind judging. What is happening is what you are doing. You do not need to ask questions or report back to yourself on what is taking place. Your feelings simply express themselves.

Learning to relax

When learning to relax using the exercises of Kum Nye, we tend to think that there is a goal, and that we must do something to achieve it. The compulsion to make an effort is always present in our minds and can become an obstacle to relaxation if we allow it to dictate the form and nature of our practice. Try not to rely on a certain form of preparation or approach to an exercise, because it will shift attention from the immediacy of the experience to the framework you have applied to what you are doing. Instead be spontaneous in your practice; approach the exercises in the way that seems most natural at the time.

In the exercises in later chapters, there are many instructions telling us how to sit still, how to breathe, how to move and massage the body. While these instructions are important

for gaining an initial feeling for each exercise, it is important to remember that there is no absolutely correct way to be or particular method for doing an exercise. If we allow the exercise instructions to dominate our practice, relaxation is impeded as we remain caught up in their external descriptions, matching outward form to the instructions given. Instead we must learn to feel our way through the exercises intuitively, letting the body lead the mind on a personal exploration as we gain awareness of the internal processes at work on an energetic level.

It is at this point, when we start to work with an internal rather than external focus, that we begin to open up and relax, without holding back. Holding back is a continuous state of waiting to be relaxed; an expectation that relaxation will come from somewhere else. When we hold back during our practice we often engage in an inner dialogue with ourselves as we comment and speculate on our apparent success or failure, our progress toward our goal of relaxation. Paradoxically, in doing so we hinder relaxation because our participation in an inner dialogue prevents us from becoming one with our bodies, from relaxing by opening to the subtle energies within us.

Rather than allowing the dialogue of your conscious mind to gain control, relax by focusing your attention on the feelings within your body and allowing the process of Kum Nye to take place. Develop an open-ended attitude – concentrate on the exercise or self-massage at hand, without worrying about results, lack of experience or a perceived need for greater effort. The more that you can do this, the fewer the distractions, thoughts and conflicts that will arise; your body will be nurtured by the increasing experience of relaxation; and your whole being will become healthier as ordinary physical energies work to release those at deeper levels of consciousness.

At the end of each exercise or self-massage, sit quietly and immerse yourself in the sensations of your body. This is an important part of your practice, an opportunity to develop and expand the feelings stimulated by each exercise. Stay with the sensations without trying to hold onto them – no effort is required. If you cling to the feelings by analyzing or categorizing them, you will interrupt the flow. Simply remain open and the energy will stimulate itself.

Building your practice

It will probably take several months before you truly learn to relax, so it is important to practise regularly. Ideally, begin by practising Kum Nye for forty-five minutes twice a day, doing sitting, breathing and movement exercises in the morning and self-massage in the evening. If you have less time to spend on your practice, set aside forty-five minutes each day and fill this time with a selection of sitting, breathing, movement and self-massage exercises. Always wait at least an hour after eating before starting your practice.

Develop your practice gradually in a balanced way. Begin by working with some of the sitting and breathing exercises, and a couple of the massages, together with a selection of the simplest gentle movement exercises. Practise these for several weeks until you sense an inner awakening to the experience of Kum Nye the development of internal awareness on a subtle energetic level. Take your time with each exercise; spend at least two or three minutes on each repetition, deepening and exploring your internal experience. If you move too quickly through the exercises you will create a false sense of progress.

As you gain confidence begin to explore some of the other exercises and massages. Chapters four to six provide a loose framework around which you can base your movement practice, although essentially you should feel free to follow your own instincts when choosing exercises – they will direct you to the exercises suitable for your needs and abilities that day.

Initially there may be times when you feel reluctant to practise, when you are unwilling to relax and feel. When this occurs, listen to your body in order to locate these feelings of resistance. As you begin your practice, focus your awareness in these areas. This will help to channel the energy released during the exercise toward the areas of resistance, melting the blockages. When you have had more experience of Kum Nye, you will come to welcome such sensations of energy in your body for they bring a renewed sense of freedom and aliveness.

With time, your body will naturally seek Kum Nye and will lead you to the exercises or variations that you most need to explore. Sometimes an exercise may happen spontaneously during your practice – not because you make a rational decision to perform that exercise, but because your feelings naturally adopt that form. When this occurs, you will develop confidence and respect for your body and a greater understanding of embodiment; you will have begun to discover your body of knowledge.

As you explore your body during the exercises and self-massages, you will probably discover sensitive and even painful areas. When this occurs breathe into the pain; then exhale slowly and gently, and relax the area. You should find that this technique, combined with the healing effect of the exercise that you are practising, transforms the pain into a deep sweetness.

If a colour or image appears during your practice, pause and look for a moment – you may have touched an experience beyond time and space, or energy centres may be opening as the process of relaxation releases tensions and blockages. At the same time you may experience an opening of your senses resulting in a heightened sensitivity to taste, colour and sound.

Your practice and others

Be confident in what you are doing and do not give up. Encourage yourself and develop an attitude of patience toward yourself and your practice. You may find that others do not support you or appreciate what you are doing, but remember that your motive for practising is not merely selfish: if we want to do our best for future generations of humanity, for our friends and family, we must begin by taking care of ourselves.

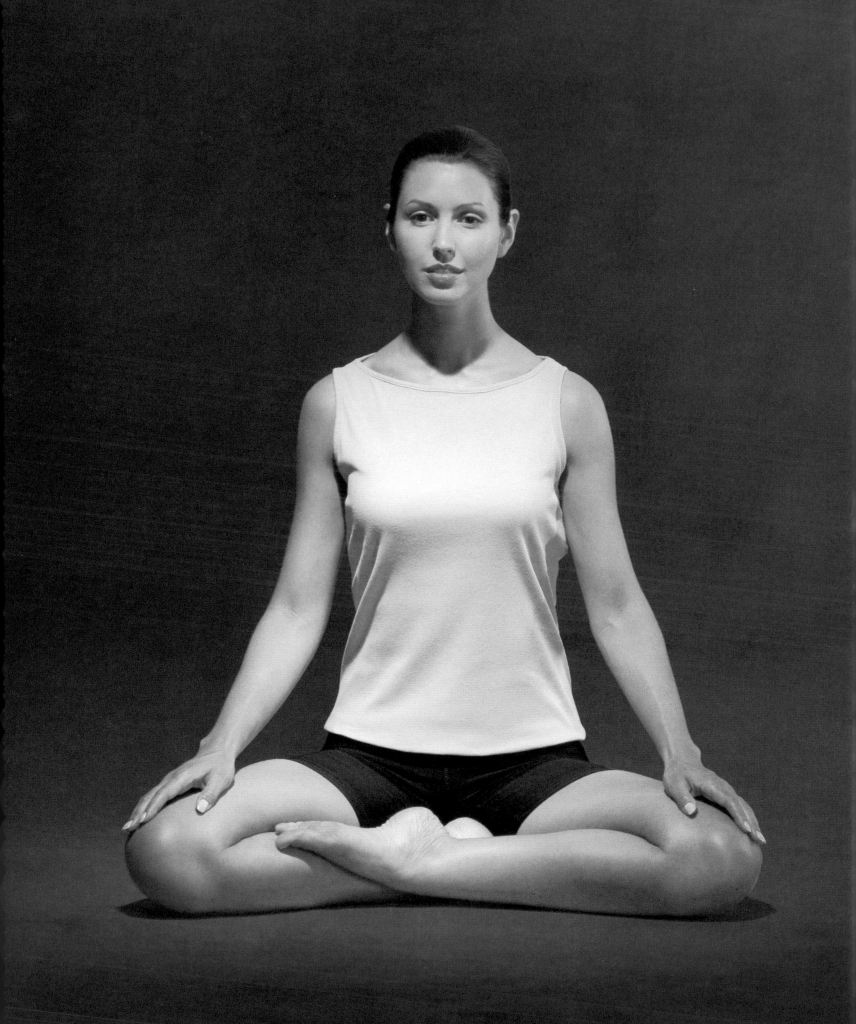

CHAPTER TWO

SITTING AND BREATHING

*"As thoughts slow down, internal harmony arises.
A sense of relief and inner sureness comes forth."*

Kum Nye begins simply, with just sitting still, relaxing and breathing. The traditional position for sitting (shown by the Buddha when he first became enlightened) is the lotus posture, which facilitates relaxation of both body and mind. Energy flows smoothly in this position and, with enough time, all mental and physical energies become transformed into positive, healing sensations. This chapter guides us through some basic sitting exercises, which encourage us to find stillness and relaxation. These are followed by a selection of breathing exercises that help us to develop slow, soft and even breathing patterns that calm and balance both body and mind. In practising these exercises we learn how to contact the energy of the breath, so that our breathing becomes an infinite source of vitality.

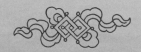

THE SITTING POSTURE

"Kum Nye begins simply, with just sitting still and relaxing."

The sitting posture and the soft, smooth breathing that it facilitates can relieve both mental and emotional agitation and physical tension. As such they provide the starting point for Kum Nye for they represent the first steps on the path toward true relaxation. Initially, you may understand relaxation in a mechanical way, believing that sitting still means that the body does not move. However, it is possible to be still without becoming rigid: as you continue to practise, you will discover that you do not need to make an effort to relax and you will eventually experience complete alertness and stillness.

The sitting posture is comprised of seven "gestures" or "aspects" (see below). The first of these is to sit with your legs in lotus, half-lotus, or simply crossed, on a mat or a cushion. If you are unused to sitting cross-legged, you may feel some discomfort initially, until you learn to relax unnecessary tension. If you feel pain in your knees, cross your legs loosely and put a higher pillow under your pelvis. The problem may be that your thigh joints are stiff. Practising the exercises opposite will help to loosen these joints.

If it is too difficult for you to sit cross-legged, sit in a straight chair with your legs uncrossed. Sit forward on the seat so that you do not lean against the back of the chair, separate your legs a comfortable distance and place your feet flat on the floor. This distributes the weight of the body on a firm triangular base.

Physical discomfort has a mental or emotional component; when our minds are not at ease, our bodies cannot be relaxed. When you feel uncomfortable while sitting, notice your state of mind. Is there an active flow of thoughts, dialogues, images and fantasies? While sitting in the sitting posture, practise the exercises on p.30 and you will find that, with time, your mind becomes calmer, the tension in your body eases and you discover a more relaxed mode of being.

THE SEVEN GESTURES

1 Sit with the legs crossed, or in half-lotus or lotus (with one or both ankles resting on top of the thigh), arranging your mat or cushion so that your pelvis is higher than your legs.

2 Place your hands on your knees, palms down. Release tension in your arms and shoulders, and relax your hands so that they rest comfortably on your knees.

3 Draw back your neck a tiny bit. Your head will move forward very slightly.

4 Ensure your spine is balanced without being rigid. This allows energy to flow naturally from the lower to the upper body.

5 Half-open your eyes and focus them loosely on the ground, following a line downward along the ridge of your nose. Your eyes should be soft and compassionate. Try to minimize blinking by relaxing the area around your eyes and moving your awareness inward.

6 Open your mouth slightly, keeping your jaw relaxed.

7 Let the tip of your tongue lightly touch the ridge of your palate, just behind the teeth. Your tongue will curve back a little.

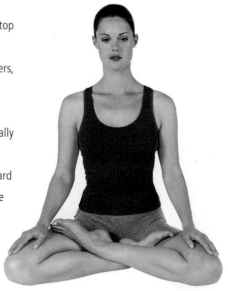

OPENING THE THIGH JOINTS

*The following two exercises help to loosen the thigh joints and can be practised
prior to the sitting posture to increase your comfort in this position.*

LETTING GO

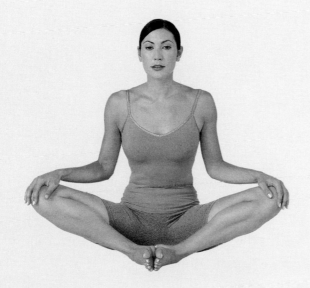

Sit on a mat or cushion with the soles of your
feet together and your hands on your knees.
Bring your feet close to your body. With your
hands pushing down on your knees, begin
a light, quick, up-and-down movement in
your legs. Focus on the upward movement.
Continue for about a minute. Then sit quietly
for a few minutes, sensing the feelings in
your body. Repeat 3 times.

MELTING TENSION

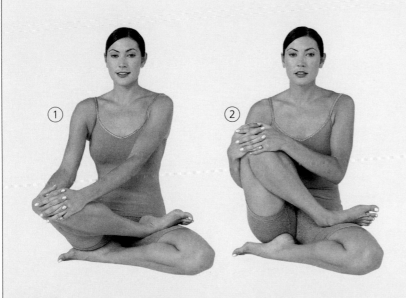

❶ Sit on a mat or cushion and cross your legs so
that your right ankle rests on your left thigh. With
your back straight, interlace your fingers and clasp
your hands around your right knee.

❷ Very slowly lift your right knee a short distance
and then lower it.

Do this 3 or 9 times, feeling the sensations in your
body. Then reverse the position of your legs and
repeat the movement 3 or 9 times. When you finish,
sit in the sitting posture for 5 minutes, allowing
your sensations to continue.

VISUALIZATION EXERCISES

These visualization exercises are performed in the sitting posture and provide the starting point for the practice of Kum Nye. "Tasting Relaxation" and "Following Sensation" offer us our first experience of Kum Nye Relaxation and teach us how to tune in to our feelings and sensations — the means by which we learn to increase our enjoyment of every aspect of living. "Expanding Feeling" helps us to broaden our feelings so that our sensory awareness is developed in a finer, more substantial way. Begin by practising "Tasting Relaxation" and "Following Sensation" together for between thirty minutes and an hour a day for one to two weeks. You can then attempt "Expanding Feeling", practising this exercise frequently over the following few weeks, daily if possible.

TASTING RELAXATION

Breathe deeply about 10 times and slowly relax your whole body. Relax your eyes, closing them if you wish, and let your mouth fall open. Let tension slip away from your forehead and scalp. Slowly sense every part of your head — your nose, ears, jaw, cheeks, the inside of your mouth — until your whole head becomes completely relaxed. Then relax the back and sides of your neck, your throat and the underside of your chin before moving to your shoulders, chest, arms and hands, belly, back, legs, feet and toes. When you find a tense place, enjoy the sensation of tension melting away. Taste the feeling of relaxation, enjoying it more and more until it nurtures every part of your body. Continue for 15 to 30 minutes.

FOLLOWING SENSATION

Sit as relaxed and still as you can. Slowly let yourself become aware of any sensation or feeling-tone that arises. You may feel a physical sensation or an emotion — this does not need to be strong, it can be light, even delicate. Tune into your inner ear. Trust in the present moment of your experience and open yourself to it. Do this in whichever way you choose. There is no right method or formulation. Whenever you feel a sensation or feeling-tone, allow it to continue for as long as possible. Continue for 15 to 30 minutes.

For the next week, allow yourself to be as relaxed as possible throughout the day. Sensitively watch your movements (even the blinking of your eyes) for subtle patterns of muscular tension. Let all aspects of your body possess a relaxed, gentle quality, including your breath, skin, hair and all your internal organs.

EXPANDING FEELING

Sit very quietly, breathing gently and evenly, with your mouth slightly open. Cast your mind back to a wonderful memory and allow it to become very real in your mind — perhaps your first love, a beautiful sunset, a scenic walk along a riverbank. Recreate the positive energy of that past time, expanding it throughout your being. Let your body heat up and your breath move a little higher in your chest, until you feel a physical sense of exhilaration. Expand the sensation throughout your body and beyond, so that you are the centre from which feelings ripple out in all directions. Now slowly draw this vital feeling back into your body. Let this energy unite and cleanse your body and mind. Continue to expand and retract your exhilarating feeling in this way for 15 to 20 minutes. If you do this whenever you have beautiful ideas, images or feelings, you will enhance your sensory awareness.

SENSATION AND BREATH

*"Once we know how to contact the energy of breath,
breathing becomes an infinite source of vitality."*

Because breathing charts the life rhythms, the way we breathe signals the disposition of our energies. When we are agitated or excited, our breath tends to be uneven and rapid; when we are calm and balanced, our breathing is even, slow and soft. This close relationship between our breathing patterns and our energies means that we can alter our mental and physical states by the way we breathe. For example, when we are very upset, we can calm and balance ourselves simply by breathing slowly and evenly.

When our breathing is consistently calm and even, the whole organism becomes balanced — physically, mentally and emotionally. As a result energy increases, health improves and quality of sleep is enhanced. This leaves the mind lucid and the body alert and sensitive so that we are more open to the richness and diversity of all levels of our experience.

The body's energy centres

The breathing of Kum Nye is a gentle form of breathing that enables us to contact the energy of the breath, which is itself inseparable from the subtle mental and physical energies that pervade the body. We can understand the energy pattern of the body by visualizing energy flowing both through and outward from the body in all directions. Located at various points down the centre of the body, from the top of the head to the base of the spine, are a number of energy centres, which include the head centre, the throat centre and the heart centre. These are termed *chakras* in the ancient Indian system of medicine and act as terminals for energy as it circulates throughout and radiates from the body. If we could see this energy pattern from a distance, it would look like a spiral, with the head centre at the top; seen from above, it would appear to be a series of concentric circles with one ring for each of the energy centres.

The energy of the breath is particularly associated with the throat centre, which both evokes and coordinates the flow of energy throughout the body. It is through the throat centre that we can most easily learn to contact and balance the energy of the breath and the other subtle energies of the body. The throat centre is traditionally pictured as a sixteen-petalled flower with two blossoms connected back to back. One eight-petalled blossom is directly linked to the head centre, the other to the heart centre; as energies pass through the throat centre, they flow outward to these other centres. When the throat centre is settled and calm, the energies flow in a balanced and coordinated way, resulting in the integration of the mind and the body.

Energy imbalances

All too often the throat centre is agitated and the energies of the body become imbalanced. When this occurs we tend to lose touch with our feelings and sensations. This in itself makes it difficult for us to move toward balance within ourselves because it breeds the sense of dissatisfaction that leads us to look outside ourselves for fulfilment.

Once in place this pattern soon becomes self-perpetuating, for the more we rely on external things to provide satisfaction and joy — be they people or material possessions — the more we lose touch with ourselves and our inner body sensations. Instead of experiencing life directly, fully assimilating our sensations and integrating them with our feelings, we get caught in patterns of thinking about our experience, labelling it and reporting back to ourselves on its nature. We thus reinforce the subject — the "I" who does the experiencing — and experience itself becomes an object, frozen in form and meaning.

When we are in this state, our feelings are actually secondary feelings, interpretations of mental images, which we then feed back to ourselves. We live predominantly in our heads, our awareness focusing on memories of past experience — mental verbalizations that are unconnected to our true feelings in the present. The flow of energy to the head centre

BASIC BREATHING EXERCISES

Before embarking upon the massage and movement exercises it is important to become familiar with these basic breathing exercises, which help us to separate out the different qualities of the Kum Nye breath. For the first week, practise soft breathing in "Joyful Breath"; for the next three or four days, explore very slow breathing in "Opening the Senses". (If you wish, spend more time on each of these exercises.) Then you can progress to "Living Life in the Breath" in which you will learn full Kum Nye breathing, which is even and balanced as well as soft and slow. This is the form of breathing that should be performed during the massage and movement exercises.

JOYFUL BREATH

Practise this breathing for 20 to 30 minutes a day for about a week. As much as you can, become aware of the quality of your breath throughout the day. Perform this exercise in the sitting posture, either on a mat or cushion, or on a straight-backed chair.

1 Sitting comfortably, make sure your mouth is slightly open, with the tip of the tongue lightly touching the palate ridge. Gently relax your throat, belly and spine and begin to breathe very softly and easily through both nose and mouth, without paying much attention to the process. This gentle breathing is quite light, yet very energizing. Let this soft breathing soothe and relax your whole being by bringing the breath to any muscle tensions in your body, and any words or images that are disturbing your mind.

2 Without trying to control the breath, let it gradually become even more calm and soft until a quality of mellowness develops. As soon as you feel a sensation – perhaps a feeling of something flowing in your throat and body – accumulate the feeling (not by trying to add anything to it, but by simply allowing it to continue). You may feel the sensation moving to different parts of your body.

OPENING THE SENSES

Practise this slow breathing for 20 to 30 minutes for 3 or 4 days. On the third and fourth days, practise twice a day if you can. When you do so, pay a little more attention to the quality of your breathing, following your breath with your awareness until you become very still.

1 Sit comfortably in the sitting posture, and begin to breathe softly through both nose and mouth. Lightly pay attention to the inhalations: gently slow them down as much as you can, while keeping the breath as soft as possible. Feel the sensations in and around your body as your inhalations slow; go deeply into these sensations, expanding and accumulating them with the breath. Continue for 10 to 15 minutes.

2 Now lightly pay attention to your exhalations: breathing out very slowly through both nose and mouth, keeping the breath light and soft, the inhalations normal. As you develop the quality of these slow exhalations, try to open your whole sensory field as much as possible – every cell, tissue and organ. Let your feelings spread like a halo throughout and around your body. Continue for 10 to 15 minutes.

LIVING LIFE IN THE BREATH

Practise this even breathing for 20 to 30 minutes every day for at least 3 months. Then continue to practise this breathing whenever you can throughout the day, whether you are working, walking or talking, and even during the night, when you awaken. Perform this breathing exercise in the sitting posture, or, as an alternative, while lying down on your back – either with your legs straight or with your knees bent and your feet flat on the floor.

1 Sitting or lying comfortably, breathe softly and slowly through both nose and mouth. Gently pay attention to your breathing, ensuring that the breath flows equally through both nose and mouth. Give equal time to inhaling and exhaling. Pay attention to the quality of your breathing: is it hard, choppy, agitated, deep? Notice how different qualities of breathing relate to different mental and feeling states, and how your mind begins to settle and feelings to flow as your breathing becomes easier and more even.

2 As you breathe, open the feeling of relaxation as wide as you can. Unite your awareness with your breath and expand any sensations that arise until you no longer know where the boundaries of your body lie; you can sense only feeling and the subtle energy that rides on the breath.

3 As superfluous muscle tensions dissolve, you will be able to penetrate different layers of feeling and you will become familiar with many subtle feeling-tones, although you may not necessarily have words to describe them. Allow these feeling-tones to expand so that they become ever deeper and more vast.

increases and the energy flow to the heart centre lessens. No longer able to contact the nurturing feelings of the heart, a sense of almost continuous dissatisfaction arises – a subtle form of anxiety felt in the throat centre as a kind of tightness, which results in the self reaching out for experience.

We experience emotional extremes when we are in this state – heightened emotions such as anger and hate, the numbing pain of severe depression and apathy. Until the throat centre settles and energy is distributed as much to the heart as to the head, we cannot truly contact our senses or touch our real feelings. Without the energy needed to activate them, our senses are unable to operate properly and seem to be asleep.

Kum Nye breathing

Kum Nye helps us to dissolve this pattern of anxiety and reaching out by leading us back to direct experience. We can begin this process by practising Kum Nye breathing, which calms the throat centre, enabling it to function smoothly. This is achieved by breathing slowly and evenly through both nose and mouth, with the mouth slightly open and the tongue lightly touching the palate. Initially this is not very comfortable, but as energy begins to travel evenly to our head and heart centres, we experience a greater sense of vitality and it becomes increasingly easy and pleasant to continue. As the flow of energies within us becomes balanced, our feelings and sensations unfold naturally and we begin to open to deep sensations of fulfilment.

When you try this form of breathing, begin by paying attention to breathing equally through both your nose and mouth. The quality of the breathing should be effortless and natural, without strain; you do not need to think to breathe correctly.

Contacting the relaxation of Kum Nye

When you breathe in this way, your body will become calm and you will begin to feel more relaxed. As soon as you notice the feeling of relaxation, taste and enjoy it. If you do not detect this feeling at first, actively evoke it by imagining your ideal of the most heavenly, exquisite feelings. In time you will be able to experience the energies of these feelings physically. Once you contact the feeling of relaxation, you have found the way.

Experience this feeling as deeply as you can; the deeper you go, the richer and more widespread the feeling will become, until it pervades every part of your body and beyond.

As the relaxation expands, develop the quality of the breath so that it becomes exhilarating. In doing so your awareness (which arises from direct experience) will gradually expand until breath and awareness are unified. When this occurs you will experience a blissful, open feeling, with a merging quality so vast it is almost overwhelming. When your feelings build to this power, they open all your energy centres, cells and senses, and your whole body becomes balanced. It is at this point that you touch the essence of Kum Nye, the pure energy of the cosmos, directly. Once this is achieved you can draw on this energy whenever you choose for it is limitless in its availability.

The union of breath and awareness

When your breath is truly balanced and unified with your awareness you can use it as a radar to detect the emotions of both yourselves and others. This awareness of the seeds of emotion and feeling enables you to balance your emotional life because it creates a space in which you can exercise conscious control of developing emotions as opposed to controlling them by blind suppression or force once they have emerged fully. Even when you find yourself in situations that arouse great anger, frustration or pain, you can dissolve the disturbance simply by being aware of your breathing and making the breath calm, slow and rhythmical. The longer you accumulate energy with the breath, the more your whole body will calm down.

Once we learn to accumulate energy in this way, we can develop this process throughout the day and night, not only during our Kum Nye practice. When this occurs our lives acquire a healthy rhythm, undisturbed by extremes. The whole body relaxes, muscular tensions and mental blockages dissolve, and energy is distributed everywhere. The exercise of tapping the energy of the breath becomes natural and effortless.

The energy of the breath is continuous with not only our internal energies, but also with the energies that pervade our environment. Consequently, in using the energy of the breath to contact our inner energies, we also succeed in contacting those in the world around us. The result is a merging of the outer world of objects and the inner world of the senses as the two become harmonized and balanced.

The breathing exercises

To reap the lasting benefits of Kum Nye breathing it is important to work continually with the breath, otherwise your body, mind and senses will slip back into an unbalanced rhythm. Try to practise the Kum Nye breathing exercises for twenty to thirty minutes every day for at least three months. You should also try to breathe in this way throughout the massage and movement exercises. After three months, continue to practise your Kum Nye breathing during the massage and movement exercises, and perform the breathing exercises whenever you feel the need to refresh your contact with the energy of the breath.

Begin by breathing very easily. As you progress, breathe more slowly, letting the breath slow down until eventually it becomes totally smooth and even, almost without inhalation or exhalation. Your energy will then steadily increase and you will gradually develop a quality of awareness akin to that of meditation. As you perform the massage and movement exercises, check your breathing from time to time to see how you are progressing toward this goal.

As you do these exercises, allow your breathing to nourish and relax you, increasing your feelings of enjoyment until they become so substantial that they are almost tangible. Let the breath bring more vitality to your body and greater clarity to your mind. Throughout the day, allow your breathing to sustain and nurture you. Experience your senses awakening, giving your life a magical, spicy flavour.

ADVANCED BREATHING EXERCISES

The advanced breathing exercises are best practised as an accompaniment to the massage and movement exercises to help reinforce our contact with the breath. Perform "Breathing OM AH HUM" in the evening before going to sleep – it provides an ideal finish to a massage session and ensures a good night's rest. Perform "Cleansing Breath" when you rise in the morning, so that you begin the day feeling relaxed and energized.

BREATHING OM AH HUM

In this exercise the mantra OM AH HUM merges with the breath. You do not actually pronounce these sounds; you are simply aware of them. OM signifies the energy of existence and hence all physical forms; AH symbolizes interaction – the energy that informs the physical form and keeps it alive; HUM represents creativity – all thoughts, awareness and activities. Together OM AH HUM symbolizes the enlightened body, mind and spirit.

1 Lie down on the floor on your back with your arms at your sides. Separate your legs about the width of your pelvis. If it feels more comfortable, support your head with a pillow and put a pillow under your knees. Open your mouth slightly and lightly touch the tip of your tongue to your palate. Breathe gently and evenly through both nose and mouth.

2 During the inhalation visualize or think about OM. Hold the inhalation slightly when you reach your maximum lung capacity and focus on the syllable AH. As you exhale, think HUM. Breathe smoothly, giving equal time to inhaling and exhaling.

3 When holding the inhalation during AH, hold in your lower stomach; as you exhale, let the breath go equally from your stomach, nose and mouth. Breathe a little heavily to start, then gradually, without effort, decrease the amount of air you take in until your breathing becomes very slow and almost silent. Be very still at the end of each breath. After a while your breath will continue in this fashion by itself. As it does so, gradually shift your attention from your body to the realm of feeling and energy, allowing your awareness to expand beyond the physical dimensions of the body. Continue for half an hour.

CLEANSING BREATH

This breathing exercise is traditionally used to rid the system of the impurities that accumulate during the night and to renew the body's energies in preparation for the new day.

1 Sit cross-legged on a mat or cushion and hold your right hand with the thumb held under curled fingers and the index finger straight. Rest your left hand lightly on your left knee.

2 Inhale deeply, taking in as much air as possible. Imagine that this breath fills every cell in your body.

3 Place the middle joint of your right index finger against your right nostril, closing it tightly. Close your mouth and exhale slowly through your left nostril as fully as possible. Continue exhaling until your stomach begins to quake. Then rest for a moment, breathing normally through both nostrils. Repeat twice.

4 Perform the exercise 3 times on the right side, resting briefly after each exhalation. Finally exhale fully from both nostrils 3 times. Then sit for a few minutes, breathing normally and enjoying the sensations in your body.

As you perform the exercise, visualize the impurities coming out of your body as a dull white stream from the left nostril, a dark red stream from the right nostril and a deep blue out of both nostrils. Imagine that you are blowing all the attitudes with which you push things away from you, such as aversion, dissatisfaction and fear, out of the left nostril, all the attitudes and emotions with which you hold onto things, such as desire and attachment, out of the right nostril, and the dull and confused quality of your everyday mind out of both nostrils.

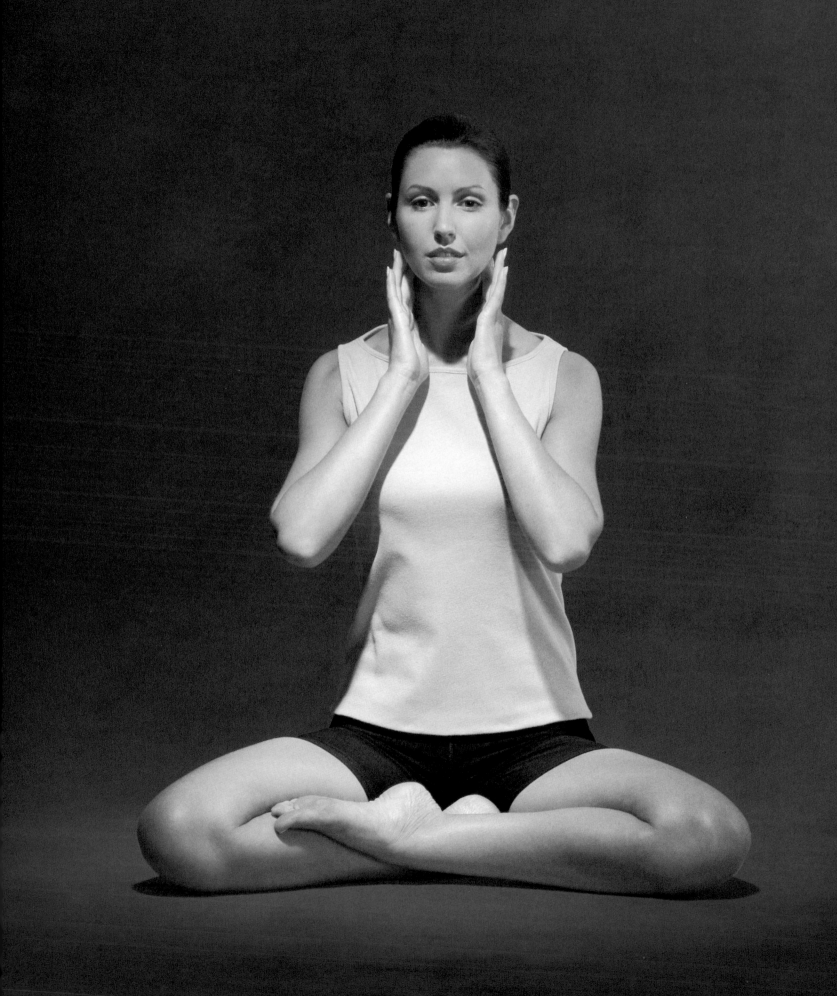

CHAPTER THREE

SELF-MASSAGE

"Our feelings and our bodies are like water flowing into water. We learn to swim within the energies of the senses."

The practice of Kum Nye integrates feelings directly with the body, instead of channelling them through the mind. Kum Nye self-massage aids this process by melting accumulated tension and gently releasing energy that has been frozen at a subtle level by our fixed attitudes and concepts. This released energy transforms into feeling experience, which then fills every cell in the body. As we live closer to the energy of feeling, we find that direct experience is far more substantial and grounded than that which is channelled through thoughts and imaginings. This chapter guides us through a series of self-massages for every part of the body. When we perform these exercises daily for at least six weeks, our feelings become more tangible, occurring not only during practice, but throughout the day.

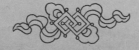

THE LANGUAGE OF TOUCH

"Our body is like a vessel filled and surrounded by space. When we touch our substance, we stimulate ourselves and the universe simultaneously. Our whole body exercises in space."

Massage means interaction. When you massage yourself, your whole body participates in the massage: a reciprocal relationship develops between your hand and the muscle or point massaged, generating feelings that stimulate interactions throughout the body. Interaction also occurs between physical and non-physical levels of existence and this interaction stimulates certain energies, which, not restricted to the body's boundaries, spread to the surrounding world.

The massage of feeling

When you begin Kum Nye massage, let go of any preconceptions or associations you may have about the practice, and move beyond the level of thoughts and concepts to the level of experience. Explore each feeling that arises in full, expanding it through your senses and thoughts. As you do so you will discover different feeling-tones, which can be explored further. Once you move inside a feeling, it will expand itself in an inner massage. Initially a feeling will bring to mind various images. At a deeper level, the feeling will be deeply nurturing, without images. Finally, you become the feeling, and there is no longer any experiencer or "I", only a sense of openness and completion.

To achieve this sense of oneness during your massage, you need to stretch the bonds of your ordinary conceptions, viewing yourself not as a individual entity comprised of separate systems, but as an integral being intimately connected to the cosmos. From this perspective, when you press a point on your body, no part of your body, and in fact no part of the universe, need be excluded. Everything becomes part of the massage.

Starting self-massage

Begin by massaging yourself for forty-five minutes or more every evening for at least six weeks. After six weeks you may want to continue with the evening massage, or alternatively you may want self-massage to be a part of your daily Kum Nye practice (in addition to the sitting, breathing and movement exercises). Although it is best done in the evening, massage can also be done at other times.

Try taking a hot shower or bath beforehand to relax your muscles and open your body to feeling. At the start of the massage, energize your hands (see opposite), then oil and rub your body in a random way. Allow your feelings to guide you to the areas that need particular attention and let them tell you when to increase or decrease pressure. Where you feel pain, rub with particular sensitivity and thoroughness, allowing the feelings and the massage to move together in rhythm. In this way, massage as much of your body as you can reach – do not neglect your arms, legs or feet.

Gradually deepen your experience of the massage, unifying breath, body, senses and mind. Breathe very slowly and lightly through both nose and mouth. This helps the breath to merge with sensation, developing a vital penetrative quality that spreads throughout the body, releasing the congested energies that inhibit the free flow of feeling. Expand feeling and sensation to encompass thoughts, so that as you rub and press, your hand becomes the eye of your mind, and your mind enters your body. At the end of the massage, sit still for five or ten minutes and feel the subtle ripples of sensation spreading outward from your body. Afterwards apply a natural perfume or, alternatively, burn some incense to prolong the process of relaxation. If you are doing the massage right before going to bed, try drinking a cup of hot milk with some honey to help you sleep.

The guided massages

After two or three evenings of "random" massage, introduce some of the specific massages detailed in this chapter, exploring two or three new techniques at a time. Initially, emphasize

ENERGIZING THE HANDS

*This massage will animate your hands. Do it at
the beginning of each massage session.*

1 Sit comfortably with your back straight, breathe gently through both nose and mouth, and relax. Oil your hands lightly. Bend your arms at the elbows and hold your hands open, with the palms up, at the level of your heart. Cup your hands a little, as if holding energy in them. Feel the sensations – perhaps tingling or warmth – in your hands and fingers. Hold the energy in your fingers; then let it pass into your hands like a flame reaching and spreading. From your hands let the energy pass into your arms, and through your arms into your heart. Allow your whole body to feel nourished by these sensations of energy. **2** Once you feel these sensations, bring your hands together and rapidly rub the back of your left hand with the palm of your right. You can do this movement quite hard and fast. Follow the sensations – you may feel energy going into your heart and neck, and into the middle of your back. Reverse the position of your hands and rub briefly. **3** Now rub your palms together rapidly until they feel hot. Once again hold your hands open, palms up, at the level of your heart, cupping them a little. Take a minute to feel the sensations flowing in your hands and body, then slowly begin your chosen massage.

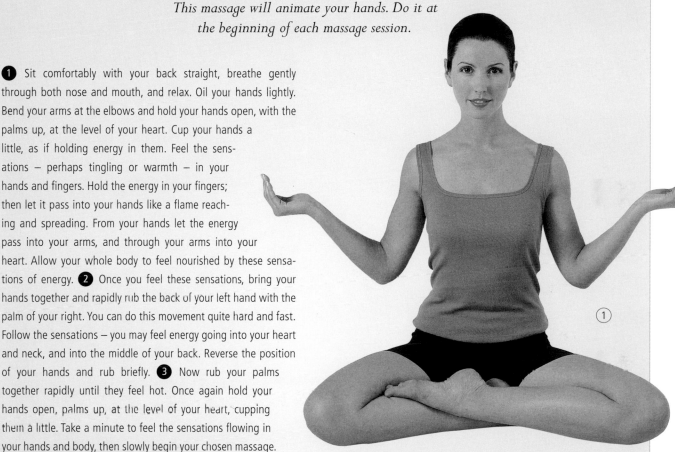

①

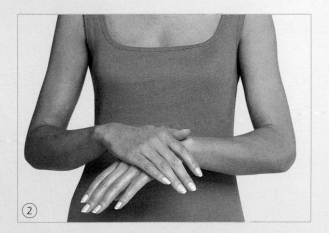

②

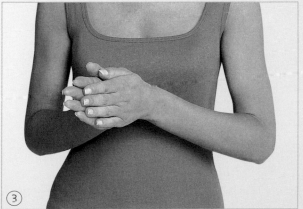

③

your upper body – your face, head, neck, shoulders and chest – but feel free to experiment. Locate points of stress and blockage and loosen them, freeing the body from its tight inner and outer harness.

A number of the massages, such as the those for the legs, the hips and the feet, specify the position that you should adopt during the massage. Where no position is indicated verbally, simply assume the position that feels most comfortable and natural to you; this may be standing, sitting on a chair, or sitting in the sitting posture (see p.28) on the floor (or on a mat or cushion if preferred).

Each time you begin a Kum Nye massage session, awaken the sensitive energies of your hands using the exercise on p.39. During the massage, bear in mind that your hand is capable of touching your whole body when it appears to touch only a part. Develop the feelings in your palms, fingers and thumbs. Whenever possible, use your whole hand to massage your body; develop reciprocity between your hand and the part that you are massaging, and be aware of subtle linkages to other parts of your body.

Throughout all of the massages, remember to breathe gently and evenly through both nose and mouth. This centres the mind within the body, sharpening awareness of the feelings and sensations stimulated during the massages. Once we have made contact with these feelings, we can begin to develop the internal energy massage of Kum Nye (see p.18).

The pressure points

Kum Nye massage is oriented toward a number of sensitive and powerful pressure points, which stimulate energy interactions throughout the body. You may find that pressure on some places has an immediate effect and on others has no noticeable effect at first. Touching certain spots may restore memories or past negativities, while others may stimulate joyful feelings. As you work to release the tension in your body, you may also release mental and emotional blockages. Once this tension melts away, only feeling or experience is left. Do not label or identify the nature of the feeling. Simply allow it to continue melting until it fills each cell with pure energy and experience.

When you are directed to work with specific acupressure points during the course of the massages, be aware of the effects that are produced by different degrees of pressure. At first press very lightly; gradually develop a medium pressure; then, when appropriate, press strongly. When you want to diminish the pressure, do so very gradually: subtly lighten the strong pressure to medium pressure, and then slowly to light pressure. In this way you will develop awareness of six distinct stages of the massage and, with more practice, you will develop additional subtleties of pressure. Above all, be careful not to release the pressure suddenly for this will shock the system, resulting in the loss of the subtle qualities of feeling. Instead, experience fully the gradual lifting up and putting down of your hand and fingers.

MASSAGE FOR THE HANDS

Massaging your hands will tune, tone up and enliven the energy of your whole body.
The hand massage is comprised of two parts: a general massage (steps 1 to 6); and a massage oriented
toward the acupressure points (steps 7 to 14). Do the complete massage on both hands.

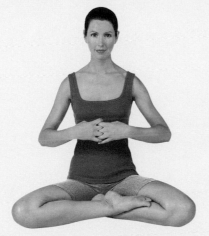

STEP 1

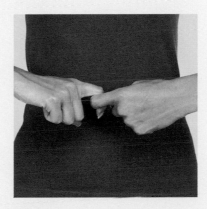

STEP 2

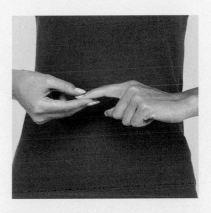

STEP 3

1 Interlace your fingers tightly with the palms and fingers toward you. Pull your hands apart under tension by squeezing your fingers together as you do so, massaging down the fingers until your hands spring apart. Repeat, feeling the sensations awakened in your body. **2** One by one, hook each finger with the corresponding finger of the opposite hand. Pull under tension until the two fingers slip apart. **3** Massage each fingertip in turn with the fingertips of the other hand. Massage down each finger from the tip to the base, working down the sides, front and back of each finger. **4** Place the base of the finger to be massaged in the web between the index and middle finger of the other hand and grasp the finger firmly.

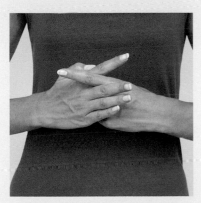

STEP 4

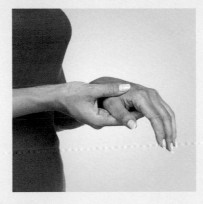

STEP 5

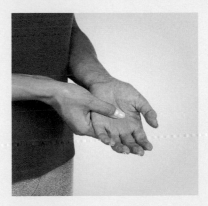

STEP 6

Slowly pull the finger while twisting it gently, moving from the base to the tip. **5** Use your thumb to work between each of the small bones (the metacarpals) on the back of your hand, massaging toward your fingers. Pay particular attention to the area between the forefinger and the thumb. **6** Massage the palm of your hand with the thumb of the other hand. You can also use the larger knuckle of the forefinger to move across the palm. Deeply massage the large mound of the thumb joint as well as the smaller mounds below the fingers. Massage between each finger. Pay attention to the small muscles between the bones, tracing them from the heel of the hand to the fingers. ▶

ACUPRESSURE POINTS
FOR THE HANDS

*The acupressure points for this and subsequent massages
are indicated by the numbered white dots.*

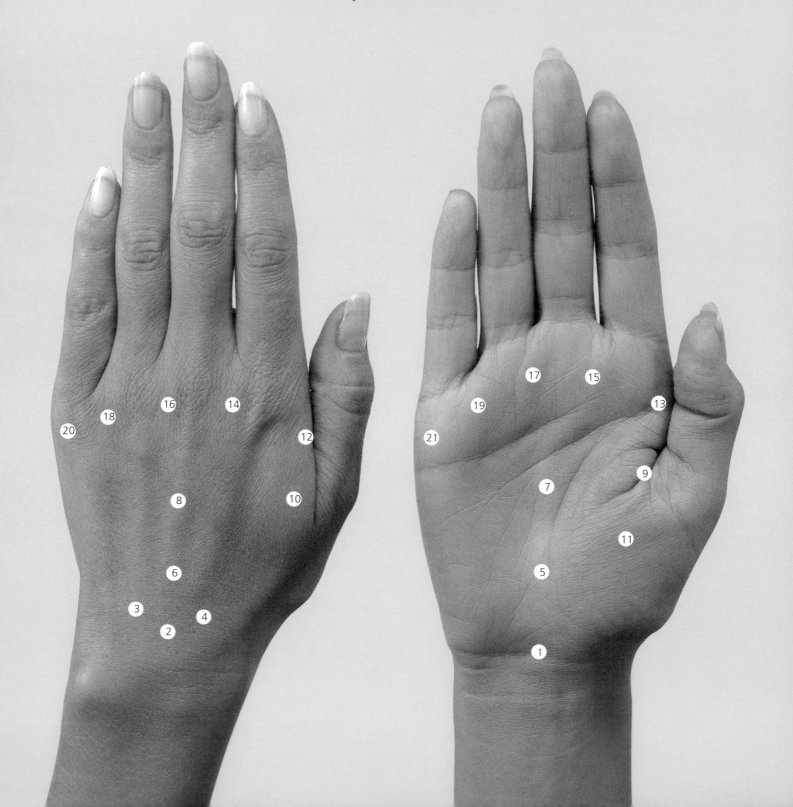

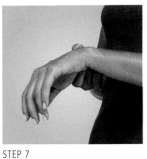

STEP 7

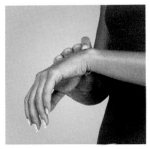

STEP 8

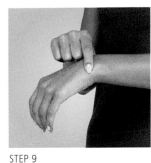

STEP 9

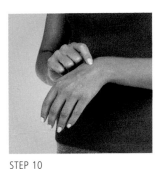

STEP 10

7 To find the first acupressure point, turn your hand palm up and look at the rings on the inside of the wrist. Place your forefinger in the middle of the ring nearest to your palm. Turn your palm down and place your thumb on the second point, on the back of your hand exactly opposite the first point. Hold your wrist tightly between your thumb and forefinger, and press strongly. Relax your chest and stomach, and any other places of tension. Breathe gently through both nose and mouth. **8** Now reverse the position, placing your forefinger on the back of your hand and your thumb on the inside of your wrist. Strongly press and manipulate the two points simultaneously. Release the pressure gradually, sensing the feelings that arise. **9** Without moving your thumb, place your forefinger on point 3, which is about a finger-width down from point 2 toward the fingers and over to the side nearest your little finger. This point lies between the bones of the little finger and the fourth finger, and may be very sensitive. Exert strong pressure with both thumb and forefinger and hold. Release slowly and gently. **10** Move your forefinger to point 4 – the corresponding point on the side of your hand nearest the thumb. Again, press strongly with thumb and forefinger and hold. You may feel strong sensations, perhaps even pain. Remain with the feelings, breathing gently through both nose and mouth. Release gradually. **11** Turn your hand palm up, measure two

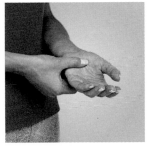

STEP 11

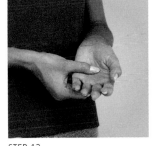

STEP 12

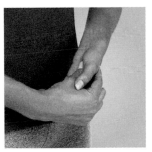

STEP 13

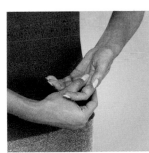

STEP 14

finger-widths toward the fingers from the first point to the fifth point, and place your thumb there. Then place your forefinger on point 6, which is on the back of your hand exactly opposite point 5. Simultaneously press these two points strongly. Release slowly, breathing evenly through both nose and mouth. **12** Place your thumb on point 7 in the middle of your palm. Place your forefinger on point 8, which is the corresponding point on the back of the hand, between the bones of the middle and fourth fingers. Press these points simultaneously, gradually increasing the pressure. Release slowly. **13** Place your thumb on point 9 near the thumb webbing and your forefinger on point 10 – the opposing point on the back of the hand. Press these two points simultaneously, sensitively increasing and decreasing the pressure. Remember to breathe gently through both nose and mouth. Now place your thumb on point 11 in the middle of the thumb mound and press and rub sensitively. The pressure can be strong. **14** The remaining ten hand points (points 12 to 21) lie in a row across the knuckles. There are five on the palm, and five on the back of the hand. Two pairs of points are at the sides of the hand, and three pairs are between the knuckle-bones. Work these points in pairs, placing your thumb on each palm point and your forefinger on the corresponding point on the back of the hand. Increase and decrease the pressure slowly. When you remove your hand from your body at the end of the massage, do so almost imperceptibly to prolong the feelings that arise.

MASSAGE FOR THE FACE

Our heads are usually busier than the rest of our bodies. Our emotions — which are closely connected to our thoughts — tend to constrict our facial muscles as well as our necks and shoulders. As you massage your face, feel the energy of released feeling move throughout your body.

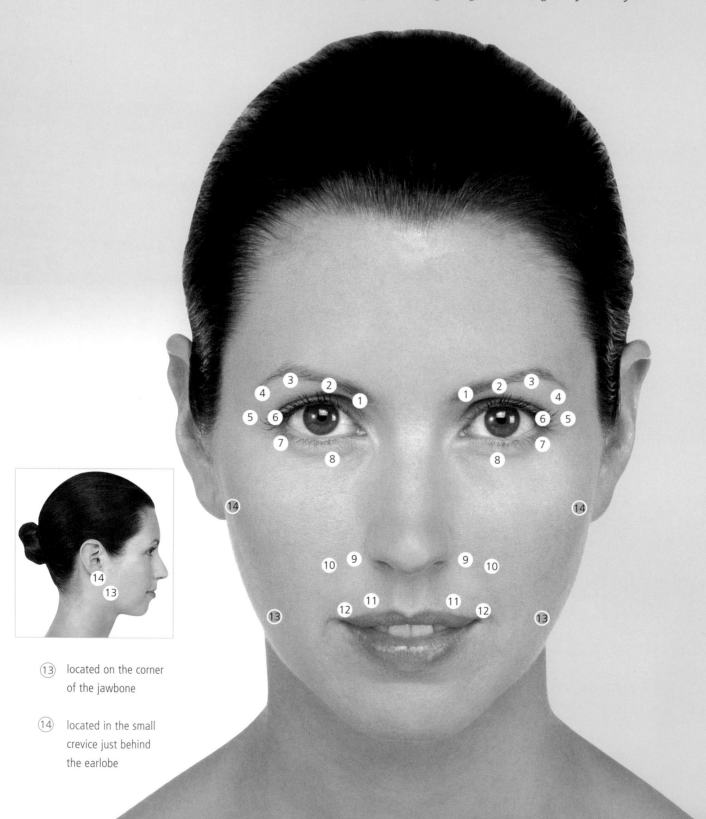

(13)   located on the corner
       of the jawbone

(14)   located in the small
       crevice just behind
       the earlobe

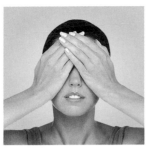

STEP 1

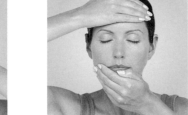

STEP 2

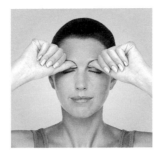

STEP 3

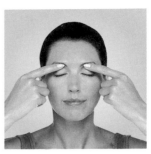

STEP 4

1 Energize your hands as described on p.39. Once your palms feel hot, place them gently over your closed eyes without exerting pressure on the eyeballs or touching your nose. Your fingers will overlap a little. Leave your hands in this position for several minutes, sensing the movement of heat and energy into your eyes and through into other parts of your body. **2** Again rub your palms together. When they feel hot, place one hand on your forehead and the other on your chin. Close your eyes and feel the flow of energy. Repeat, reversing the position of your hands. **3** Massage around the orbit of both eyes simultaneously, touching each point firmly and gently. Begin at the inner upper edges of the eye sockets and use your thumbs to find a notch in the bone beneath each eyebrow (points 1). Press up, gradually increasing the pressure, and hold. Keep your head erect. Close your eyes and go into the feelings. Release the pressure gradually, and stay with the feelings that are produced. **4** With your first or middle fingers, trace under the upper ridge to the next pair of notches (points 2), and press and massage them gently. Try closing your eyes as you do this. Trace under the upper ridges to the third pair of notches, near the arch of the eyebrow. Spend extra time here, pressing and massaging with your first or middle fingers. Experiment with different degrees of pressure. **5** At the upper outside corner of each eyesocket there is another place

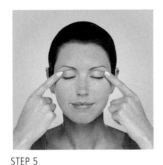

STEP 5

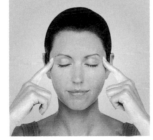

STEP 6

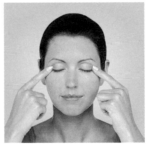

STEP 7

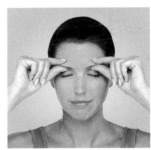

STEP 8

that deserves special attention (points 4). Use the tip of your first or middle finger to locate and massage this small crater in the bone. **6** Follow the curve of the eyesocket down to a little bump in the bone, a finger-width from the corner of the eye (points 5). Press with your forefingers, varying the pressure gradually. **7** Use your forefinger to move just inside the corner of the eyesocket to the sixth point. Press gently, breathing softly through both nose and mouth. Trace with your forefingers a short distance to the seventh point, just inside the eyesocket, a little below the sixth point. Press gently. Follow the lower curve of the eyesocket to a notch in the bone below the centre of the eye (points 8). Press gently, giving particular care to the area where the lower eyesocket meets the bone of the nose. **8** Hold your eyebrows between thumb and forefinger, at the inner edge. Press your thumbs up a little so that they rest against the bone, giving support from below. Lightly squeeze the eyebrow between thumb and forefinger and rub slowly back and forth with the forefinger. Work to the outer edge of the eyebrow; then return to the inner edge and repeat the massage. **9** With your middle fingers, press and rub the depression in the temples using a circular motion. When you find a sensitive spot, move even more slowly. Press very lightly at first, and gradually increase the pressure. Release the pressure very slowly. Then change the direction of the circles, and continue to massage, letting your feelings guide your rhythm and pressure. **10** Place the fingers of both hands side by side on the left side of the forehead. Slowly draw your hands horizontally across your forehead, bringing as much of your hand in contact with your ▶

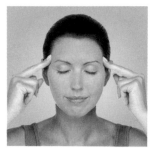

STEP 9

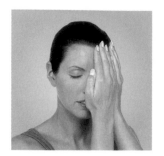

STEP 10

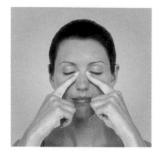

STEP 11

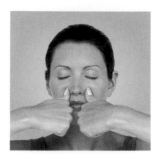

STEP 12

forehead as you can. Move back and forth several times. **11** Using one, two or all of your fingers, massage down the sides of your nose. Begin on either side of your nose near the corners of your eyes and rub with an up-and-down motion. Move slowly, varying the pressure. Pay special attention to the areas where the bone of your nose ends (about halfway down your nose), where your nose flanges meet your cheek, and where your teeth begin, below your nose (points 11). At these places press your fingers in deeper and rub slowly back and forth. Pay attention to any feelings that are released. When you finish rubbing at the base of your teeth, begin to move upward again, massaging around the nose as before. Do

this complete movement two or three times. **12** Press your thumbs in at the corner where your nose flanges meet your cheek. Your hands will hang down in front of your chin. **13** Slowly rotate your hands until your fingers point toward the ceiling. Pressing strongly, very slowly rub your thumbs back and forth across the area just below your cheekbones, out to the sides of your face. The movement of your thumbs is quite subtle although the pressure is strong. Follow the line of the cheekbones up to the bony ridges near the ears. Allow your sensations to expand, releasing subtle tensions under the skin. **14** With your forefingers, press points 9 on either side of the nose. Gradually increase the pressure, breathing evenly through

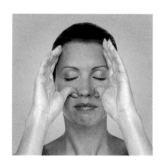

STEP 13

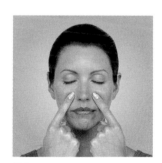

STEP 14

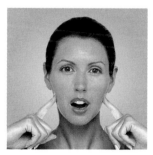

STEP 15

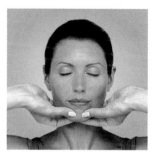

STEP 16

both nose and mouth and allowing your sensations to expand. Then follow the line of the cheekbones away from the nose to points 10, just past the curve. Again, press strongly, gradually increasing and decreasing the pressure. **15** Slowly massage across your cheeks to the points on the corners of the jawbone (points 13). Press gently with your forefingers, yawn a little, and slowly move your elbows out to the sides to open your chest. Continue to press, yawn and open your chest a little more. Relax your belly and keep your breath slow and gentle. Then slowly let your elbows come forward and release the pressure. **16** Place your fingers under your jaw and rest your thumbs on your chin with your elbows pointing out to the sides. Using all the fingers at once, press strongly under the jawbone and work thoroughly along the whole jawline, remembering to release the

pressure slowly. You will also be able to press along the top of the jawbone with your thumbs. Breathe gently through nose and mouth as you press. **17** Place your thumbs under your jaw, near the throat, resting your fingertips on your chin. Open your mouth slightly and gently press your thumbs up under the jaw. Manipulate this whole area with your thumbs, especially near the root of the tongue and the tonsils. Create a dialogue between your thumbs and these neglected muscles and try to bring this area alive. The musculature of the jaw often holds habitual patterns of thought and behaviour, and massage here may release many different feelings. Relax into whatever feelings appear as you press. At the same time, use your fingers to massage along the upper line of the jaw. **18** Smile and manipulate the corners of your smile with your thumbs. You will discover

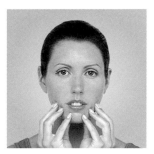

STEP 17

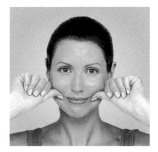

STEP 18

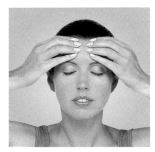

STEP 19

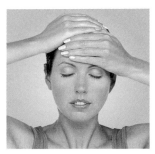

STEP 20

habitual muscle tightenings, which you can relieve with this massage. As you rub, you may also be able to massage the gum and the base of some upper teeth through the skin. When you finish rubbing, very slowly release the pressure. How does your face feel? **19** At this point in the massage, when you have covered all of the major areas of the face, it is especially pleasurable to massage the whole face in a slightly different way. Begin by massaging up the centre of your forehead and across the forehead to the temple areas. Then massage from the bridge of your nose across the cheeks toward the ears. Massage across your face from the area under the nose to the ears. Massage around your mouth, feeling the bone structure beneath your skin. Press points 11 and 12 with your forefingers. Massage across your face from the mouth, deeply manipulating the chewing muscles. Massage along the edge of the chin to the angle of the jaw. **20** Place one hand across your forehead and the other hand directly above it on your head, with the fingers of each hand pointing in opposite directions. Simultaneously move both hands slowly in the directions that the fingers point; then slowly move them back. Continue rubbing back and forth in this way, slowly moving your hands down your face to your chin, then back up again to your forehead. Your hands should be in as much contact with your face as possible. **21** Place one hand across your forehead and the

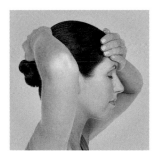

STEP 21

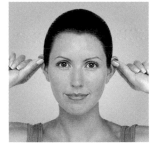

STEP 22

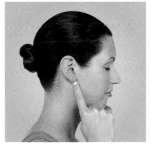

STEP 23

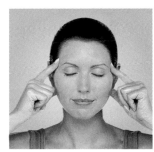

STEP 24

other hand across the back of your head. Slowly move your hands in opposite directions, one across your face, the other across the back of your head; then move them back. Your head should remain motionless during the massage. As you continue, lower your hands until you have massaged your whole head and neck. **22** Use your thumbs and forefingers to massage your ears. Start at the outer edge of the ear and gradually work toward the centre in a spiral movement. Manipulate and massage each tiny section, breathing softly and evenly through nose and mouth, merging breath and feeling. If your ears become hot, gently stop. **23** Just behind the earlobe there is a small crevice. Close your eyes and with your forefingers, press and rub near the tops of the crevices (points 14), very carefully and sensitively, without much pressure. You may feel a connection with your nostrils. Close your mouth and continue to rub very slowly and not too strongly while inhaling through the nose. Bring whatever sensations you feel into the massage. As you continue to press and rub, inhale a little more through the nose, flaring your nostrils and relaxing your lower body. Keep your back straight. Rub more and more slowly, feeling the sensations in your body, until finally you come to a stop. **24** Now place your thumbs on points 14, press lightly and, with your forefingers, slowly rub your temples in circles, first in one direction, and then in the other. Breathe softly and evenly through both nose and mouth, and as you rub, let the breath accumulate sensation and distribute it to every cell of your face, head and body. To finish, massage your face all over, paying special attention to what is bone and what is not.

MASSAGE FOR THE HEAD

*Usually we are more aware of our faces than of the rest of our heads. But the head has sensitive areas
and points that can relieve subtle blockages throughout the body, gently awakening the senses.*

The dots numbered here represent the acupressure points used in certain sections of the head massage. Points 1 to 6 fall on a midline over the top of the head, running from front to back. Points 7 to 16 are found to the sides of points 2, 4, 5 and 6. With a few exceptions, the points are four finger-widths apart.

Before attempting the head massage, gently explore these points until you become familiar with the feelings that they stimulate. Do not neglect any of the side-points. As you rub and press them, breathe slowly and evenly through both your nose and mouth, unifying breath and sensation. Go deeply into the feelings stimulated at each point, paying particular attention to the variations in sensation that are produced by different degrees of pressure. Take your time as you release the pressure, sensing the subtle flavours of feelings that develop. Once you are familiar with the points, you may want to develop the longer massages, such as those for points 3 and 6 (steps 6 and 10 respectively).

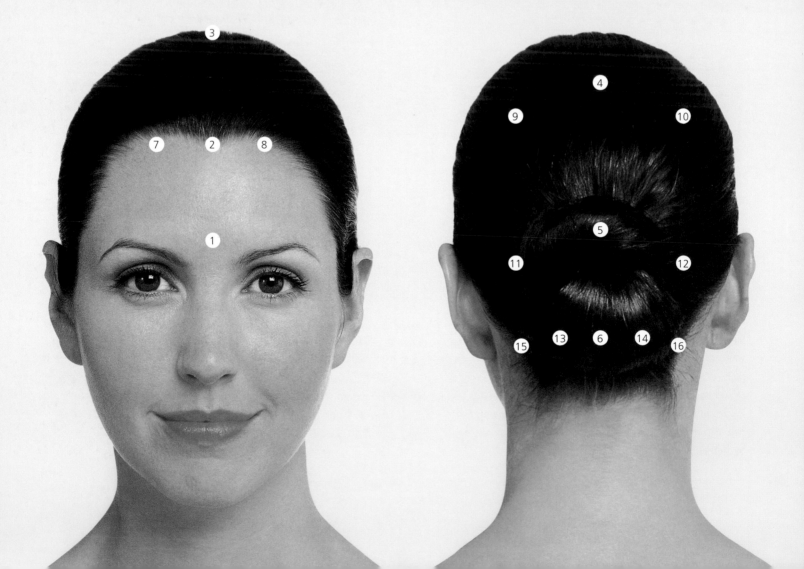

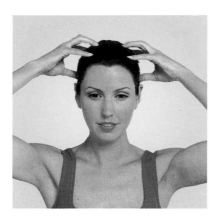

STEP 1

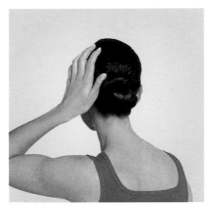

STEP 2

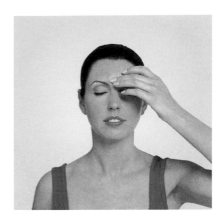

STEP 3

❶ Massage your scalp with all your fingertips. Separate your fingers and place the fingertips firmly on the front of the scalp with the thumbs on the sides of the skull. Keeping the fingertips in place, massage back and forth so that the scalp moves across the skull. Try this massage at different tempos. Touch every part of your scalp, moving from the front to the centre of the back of your head. ❷ Starting at the top of your head, trace the muscles down the left side of the back of your scalp to your neck, using all of the fingers of your left hand. Then use your right hand on the right side of the scalp. Keep your head straight as you do this. Spend extra time at places of pain or pleasure. ❸ Measure four finger-widths up from the tip of your nose to find point 1 (commonly called the "third eye"). To do this, place the fingers of your right hand on your nose so that the little finger rests on the tip and the forefinger is near the eyebrows. Keep your fingers close together and straight. The point is just beyond the forefinger. When you put pressure on this point you may feel a slight depression and a special sensitivity, which indicates the right spot. Place your middle finger

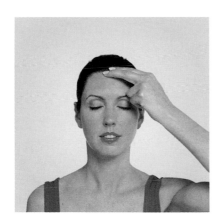

STEP 4

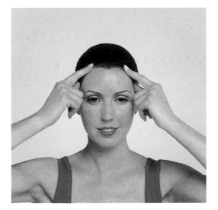

STEP 5

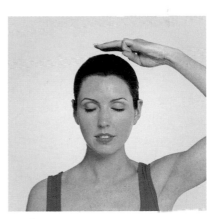

STEP 6

on this point and rub straight up about an inch (2.5cm) and then down again, exerting some pressure. Close your eyes and look inside in a relaxed way, concentrating on the point. Breathe gently through your nose and mouth. When you sense a kind of energy, transmit layers of this feeling to the centre of your body. Once you feel the energy there, slowly distribute the feeling from the centre outward to your whole body, letting it become part of every muscle. After about two minutes, let the rubbing subside gently and sit quietly with your hands on your knees, continuing to sense the feelings that have been produced. Tension is closely related to the process by which our minds produce images. Rubbing this place relieves much of that tension and stimulates the senses so that feelings begin to spread throughout the body. Body awareness and mental awareness merge, united with the breath. As this relaxation deepens, the ideas and images we produce become more balanced and vital, and of more benefit to others, for our bodies and minds are sustained from within, and we are able to be more truly caring to everyone. ❹ Pressing points 2, 7, and 8 ▶

will help to release muscle tension throughout your body. To find point 2 measure four finger-widths upward from point 1. With the first and middle fingers of one hand, press this point, and without lifting your fingers, massage one inch (2.5cm) above the point and then back down again. Repeat several times. ❺ Massage points 7 and 8, which are an inch (2.5cm) to either side of point 2, using both forefingers. Then again massage point 2. Alternate pressure on point 2 and points 7 and 8 for several minutes. ❻ To find point 3 measure four finger-widths up from point 2. This is the healing centre of the body, and the gate through which consciousness passes when we die. Through massage and visualization, we

can open this centre and learn to heal ourselves. With three fingers draw a circle at this point, rubbing and pressing lightly. As you rub, visualize a circle two inches (5cm) in diameter. Close your eyes and slowly lift up your fingers, touching your hair softly. Very slowly raise your fingers higher, two or three inches (5 or 7.5cm) above this point, and then slowly lower them. Continue to lift and lower your fingers until you feel something, perhaps an open or a cool feeling. Do not be concerned if you do not feel anything at first. Just continue to concentrate loosely on this point while sensing with your fingers. Later it may be possible to feel a little energy there when rubbing with only one fingertip. Once you are able to visualize a circular

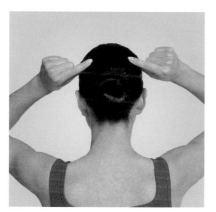

STEP 7

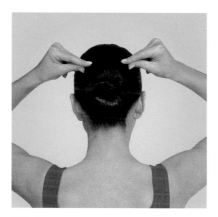

STEP 8

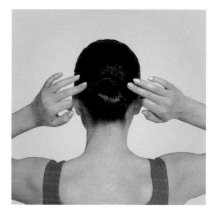

STEP 9

opening on the top of your head, visualize this circle extending into an open column from the top of your head to the base of your torso. When you are able to clearly visualize the open column within your body, visualize sparkling, white, universal energy pouring into it. This beautiful, white energy slowly fills the column, flowing down into your throat, heart and navel areas, reaching to the very root of your body. The energy is inexhaustible; it comes from all directions at once, moving like a spiral around a core. When you practise this visualization for forty-five minutes a day for one week, you may be able to feel the special joyful quality of this healing energy. If you do not contact this feeling at first, try to imagine it, and in time you will feel it. When you do, you will no longer see your body – only beautiful, white energy filling the open column like milk in a pure crystal glass. Each cell and molecule takes in this healing energy until it is completely saturated. ❼ Measure four finger-widths back from the middle of point 3 to find the fourth point. From here measure four finger-widths down on each side of the head to find points 9 and 10. Again, a special

feeling, almost of pain, indicates the right places. Concentrate on the side-points rather than on the fourth point itself. Close your eyes and rub and press point 9 with your left thumb and forefinger, and point 10 with your right thumb and forefinger. Whatever you feel, allow yourself to actually become that feeling, and go with it wherever it goes. Release the pressure gradually, breathing evenly through both nose and mouth, and allowing your sensations to be distributed throughout your body. ❽ Hold the scalp muscle tightly between thumb and forefinger and rub up and down an inch (2.5cm) from the middle of each point. Rubbing these points vigorously will loosen tension in the neck muscles. ❾ To find point 5 measure four finger-widths down the back of the head from the fourth point. To locate points 11 and 12, measure four finger-widths down on each side of point 5. Focus initially on points 11 and 12. With your eyes closed, rub these two points slowly with your middle fingers, breathing softly through both nose and mouth. As you rub and press, bring breath, mind, fingers and sensation so close together that you are no longer sure if you are being massaged by hand, mind, feeling or breath. Let your awareness and your breath enrich your sensations until they become so full and open-ended that they spread beyond your body, stimulating nurturing interactions in the world around you. **10** Point 6 is the most important of the head points. It is located at the back of the neck near the juncture of the skull and the spine, approximately four finger-widths from the centre of the fifth point. It may be a little difficult to find at first – it is not in the same place on everyone. If you cannot find it initially, you will find it another time, particularly if you work regularly with the pressure points on your head and face. You can approach this point by rocking your head gently back and

forth, with your eyes closed. Support your forehead with one hand, and with two or three fingers of the other hand press at the back of your neck near the base of the skull. The spot you are looking for can be anywhere within two or three inches (5 or 7.5cm) of the top of the spine. Perhaps you will find an edge or corner that will lead you to a very sensitive area. You may feel a tiny cracking inside. There is a special energy at this point, a deep kind of pain that is easily transformed into pleasure. Sometimes it seems like an extremely delicious feeling. When your rubbing produces any special or strange feeling, then you have found the right place. Expand this feeling as much as you can. Inhale a little more deeply, and let the

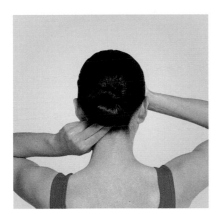

STEP 10

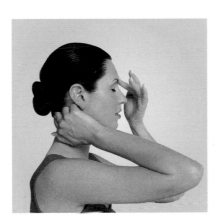

STEP 11

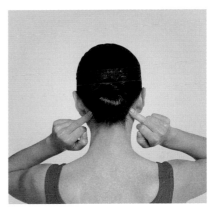

STEP 12

exhalation flow gently. Discontinue rocking your head, but continue to manipulate the point; work with it as if it had four corners, each of which you can press and rub. Relax your belly, and let your body be still and calm. Imagine that you are flying and that your body is light and airy. Go deeply into the feeling. Sometimes this feeling can be so deep and sensitive that you feel you want to cry. Distribute the feeling all the way down your spine to the sacrum. This deep feeling brings all of the subtle senses alive. Many tensions become caught in this place and rubbing it refreshes all bodily energies. Feeling washes through the spine and the backs of the shoulders, sometimes reaching the heart. **11** Simultaneously rub and press point 1 and point 6, concentrating lightly on the sixth. It does not matter if you cannot find the the sixth point exactly. Even if the two points are not connected in a direct line, pressing these two areas simultaneously relieves various sensitive blockages. Close your eyes, and rub the two points strongly with equal pressure for about thirty seconds. Then release the pressure slowly, sit very still, and concentrate loosely on the back of your

head and neck. Feel the energies moving through your forehead, perhaps above the eyeballs, to the back of your head and spine. If you do not feel anything, tighten the eyeballs a little, keeping your eyes closed. Then slowly loosen them, and notice any sensations in the back of your neck or head. There may be a sensation of heat, or a warm and blissful feeling. Sometimes you can almost feel the neck muscles becoming warm and light. Feel it more, concentrating loosely on the back of your neck and sensing the feelings flowing down your spine and perhaps into your heart. If you want to develop this particular massage, practise it for forty-five minutes a day for at least two weeks. If possible, practise twice a day. **12** Points 13 and 14 are approximately one inch (2.5cm) either side of point 6, along the base of the skull. Use your middle fingers and gradually develop strong pressure as you rub these points. Points 15 and 16 are approximately one inch (2.5cm) from points 13 and 14, toward the ear and down a little, near the tip of the mastoid process. Use your middle fingers to experiment with different degrees of pressure on these points.

MASSAGE FOR THE NECK

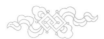

You can do this neck massage, or portions of the massage, at various times during the day whenever you feel tense. As your neck becomes more relaxed, your head and heart will become more integrated and you will experience feelings more intensely.

Difficult situations always seem to catch us when there is the least time to deal with them. Tension builds up, often settling in the neck and in the musculature where the neck meets the shoulders and head. When feeling especially tense, notice if you are holding tension in your neck. If so, try to relax for a few minutes. Slowly begin to rub your neck, pressing lightly at first. Visualize soothing feelings spreading from your neck down through your spine into all your limbs and up into your head. These feelings will lighten your whole body and ease tension in your mind so that you can think more clearly. When the mind and body are relaxed, both function better, problems take care of themselves, and the days seem lighter and easier.

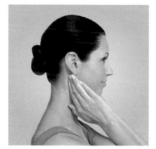

STEP 1

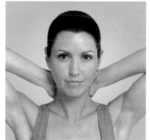

STEP 2

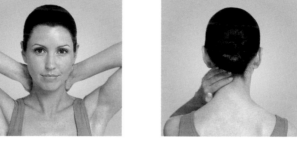

STEP 3

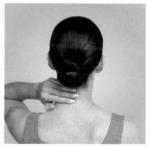

STEP 4

❶ With your middle fingers, find the bumps in your skull behind your ears, and begin to stroke down the neck muscle. You may want to use two fingers. Stroke, rub, and press down this muscle (the sterno-mastoid) following it down your neck to your shoulder. Near the shoulder, the muscle separates into two strands. See if you can locate this separation, trying to widen it as you massage. Press this point with your middle fingers, increasing and decreasing the pressure. Continue massaging the sterno-mastoid muscle for at least ten minutes, experimenting with differ-ent hands and degrees of pressure, remembering always to release the pressure slowly. ❷ Press the sterno-mastoid muscle between your thumb and four fingers, working up and down the muscle in this way. Then clasp your hands behind your neck and knead this muscle with the heels of your palms. Breathe softly and evenly through both nose and mouth as you massage, allowing the gentle influence of the breath to permeate the tensions in your muscles and mind, releasing nurturing feelings. ❸ Using the first and middle fingers of your left hand, slowly knead, press and stroke down the muscles along the left side of the back of your neck. Then

use your right hand to do the same for the muscles on the right side of the back of your neck. ❹ With the index or middle finger of one hand, press just above the large vertebrae at the base of the neck. (There is a large bump there on a line with the shoulders.) Slowly move your head back and press the point strongly. Release the pressure gradually. Then move your head forward and again press the point strongly. Release the pressure slowly, breathing gently. Slowly lift your head. ❺ Massage the left side of the back of your neck with your left hand, stroking in from the sides toward the centre-back of your neck in a slightly upward direction. Repeat on the right side with your right hand. Keep your head up and your chin in as you do this. ❻ This is a turning movement from the front of the neck to the back. Place your right hand under your chin with the heel of your hand near the hollow of your throat and the fingers and thumb curving around the right side of your neck. Keep your chin up. Slowly glide your right hand around to the right toward the centre-back of your neck with your whole palm and fingers touching your neck and your thumb and fingers together. As your right hand moves around your neck, place your

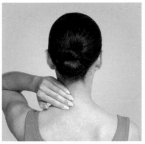

STEP 5

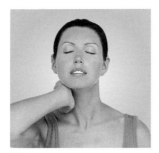
STEP 6

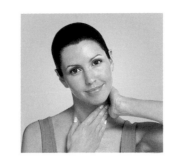
STEP 7

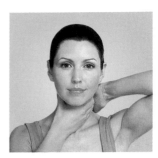
STEP 8

left hand under your chin, thumb and fingers together pointing to the right, and follow the path of the right hand. As you complete the turning movement with the left hand, begin again with the right. Continue the movement until it becomes smooth. Then repeat the action on the left side of your neck. **7** Bend your head so your right ear moves toward your right shoulder. With your fingers pointing up, pass first your left and then your right hand, across the left side of your neck along a line from the base of your throat, just above the breast bone, to the area just behind the ear; and along the base of your skull to the centre of the back of your head. Continue this massage for several minutes, developing a smooth and steady stroking motion with your hands. As you stroke breathe gently and evenly through both nose and mouth. Then bend your head toward your

left shoulder and continue the massage on the right side of your neck. **8** In this movement you alternate between massaging your throat and the back of your neck. Taking a firm hold, encircle the base of your throat with your right hand, thumb and fingers on either side of the throat. Place the left hand on the back of your neck, thumb and fingers together, the heel of your hand on the left side of the neck and your fingers curved around to the right side. Begin the massage by stroking slowly up your throat with the palm and fingers of your right hand. Lifting your chin, stroke up your throat and under your chin until your hand moves off the edge of your jawbone. As you do this, support your head with your left hand. **9** Return your right hand to the base of your throat and support your head from the front as you stroke up the back of your neck with your

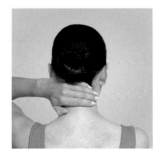
STEP 9

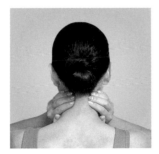
STEP 10

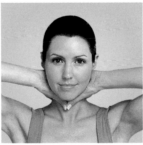
STEP 11

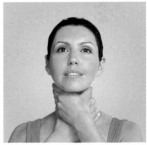
STEP 12

left hand. Your head will bend forward as you stroke. Continue just past the base of the skull and then return your left hand to the base of your neck and begin to stroke up your throat with the right hand once more. The massage should be soft and gentle. Allow yourself to feel the sensations generated throughout your whole body. Do the complete stroke at least three times. **10** Place your hands at the back of your neck along the base of the skull with your fingers pointing toward each other. Using the thumbs and fingers, slowly stroke across the muscles, moving out from the spine to the sides of your neck. Press strongly as you stroke. When you reach the sides, return your hands to your spine and repeat the movement further down. By the third time you should have covered the entire length of your neck. Continue the massage for several minutes, breathing gently through

both nose and mouth as you expand your feelings and sensations. Relax your belly and the area around your eyes. **11** Place both hands around your neck with the thumbs under your chin and your fingers at the back of your neck. Stroke down the length of your neck, with as much contact between the hands and neck as possible. Continue for at least one minute. **12** Place your right hand under your chin with the thumb and middle finger on the muscles on either side of your throat and the rest of your hand in as much contact with your neck as possible. Open your mouth slightly, and lift your chin a little. Very slowly stroke down your neck. Begin to stroke with your left hand as soon as there is room under your chin so that the second stroke begins before the first one ends. Continue, alternating hands for several minutes, breathing gently through both nose and mouth.

MASSAGE FOR THE SHOULDERS

Our shoulders are often tense with unexpressed feelings. When we gently release these tensions,
feeling flows more smoothly between the chest and neck, and between the front and back of the body.
If you are pregnant or have had any kind of neck injury,
omit the head rotation in this massage.

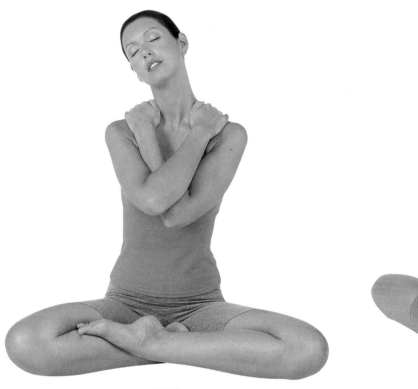

STEP 1

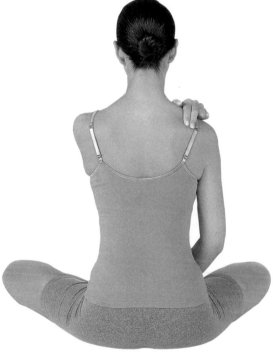

STEP 2

❶ Cross your arms and rest your hands on the opposite shoulder, close to your neck. Keeping your hands in this position, use your middle fingers to massage your shoulder muscles in a circular movement. Move the fingers very slowly, pressing strongly. As you do this, very slowly rotate your head clockwise, with your eyes closed, breathing softly through both nose and mouth. Coordinate the two movements. After three clockwise rotations, make three counterclockwise rotations. Remember to move very slowly and to breathe gently and evenly through both nose and mouth. Release the pressure slowly as the rotations come to an end. Then sit quietly for a few minutes.

❷ Press with the middle and index fingers of one hand on the back of the opposite shoulder, where the bone of the shoulder blade divides. As you press, slowly rotate the shoulder in first one direction, then the other, gently breathing through your nose and mouth. Increase and decrease the pressure gradually. Repeat the massage on the other shoulder. Now massage the trapezius muscle, which covers the shoulder and upper back. Work over the top of your shoulders and down the shoulder blades, moving toward the spine and then back up to the top of the shoulders; slowly massage any knots and tender areas until they become more relaxed. Spend at least ten minutes on this massage.

MASSAGE FOR THE CHEST

Massaging the chest improves breathing and circulation, and helps to open the heart to feeling.
This massage is particularly appropriate for women, who frequently hold tension in this area.

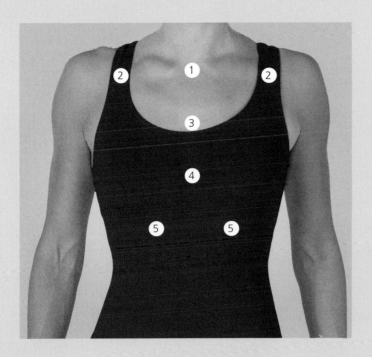

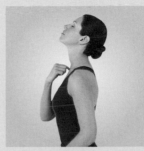

STEP 1

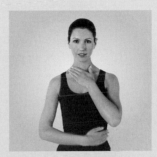

STEP 2

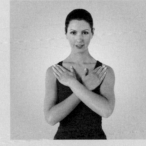

STEP 3

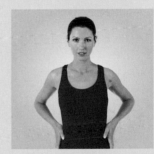

STEP 4

Using one or two fingers, slowly press along the collarbone from the base of your neck to your shoulder. Then press along and between each rib from the breastbone to the sides of your chest and under your arms. Work thoroughly in a meditative way, breathing into the areas that you are massaging. Pay particular attention to points 1 to 5. (Point 1 is just above the breastbone; point 4 lies midway between the nipples; and point 3 is halfway between points 1 and 4.) **1** Press point 1 with your index finger or thumb and, as you do so, arch your spine and neck backward without straining. Do not let your head go all the way back. Hold for a minute, continuing to press strongly. Breathe gently through both nose and mouth. Very slowly release the pressure and straighten your spine and neck. **2** Now massage the chest and the belly. Place your left hand at the base of your throat, thumb and fingers on either side of the throat, and place your right hand on the left side of your waist. Make sure both hands are in full contact with your body. Very slowly and firmly, simultaneously glide your left hand down over your chest and belly to your left waist, and your right hand up your belly and chest to the base of your neck. Your hands will

move along parallel paths, in opposite directions. Then in the same way, move your right hand down to the left side of your waist as you move your left hand up to the base of your throat. Continue this massage for several minutes, developing a steady rhythm and paying attention to any feelings that arise. Join your feelings to the breath; then bring them into the massage and let them deepen the quality of the rhythm. Then continue the massage for several minutes on the right side of your body. **3** Place your right hand near the top of your left shoulder and your left hand near the top of your right shoulder. Keeping both palms in contact with your chest, move your hands toward each other and then away from each other, slowly and rhythmically, until you have covered the entire surface of your chest. Continue for at least one minute, breathing gently through nose and mouth. **4** Place your hands flat on the sides of your body, fingers pointing down. Pressing firmly, slowly move your hands down your sides to your hips. The contact between your hands and your body should be as full as possible. Breathe softly through both nose and mouth. Continue for several minutes.

MASSAGE FOR THE BELLY

When the belly truly relaxes, we become free from grasping. Massage here is especially important for men because it is common for men to hold tension in this area. When you are away from home, perhaps in a tense or emotional situation that is giving you difficulty, the stomach massage can be particularly helpful. You may find that it produces feelings of deep relaxation, which flow outward from your stomach, affecting your whole outlook, enabling you to think clearly and act effectively. What appeared to be unpleasant may even become enjoyable. This massage is best done in the evening, at least one hour after eating, without clothes.

1 Lie down on your back with your eyes closed. Separate your legs a comfortable distance, bend your knees and draw your feet toward your body a little. Relax your belly.

STEP 1

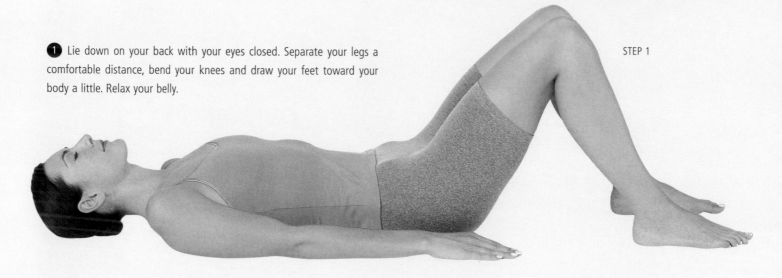

2 Place your right hand on your lower belly and your left hand on your upper belly. Let the contact between your hands and your belly be as full as possible. Slowly begin to massage in a large circle, moving your right hand up on the right side of your belly and your left hand down on the left side. When the left hand crosses over the right arm, let the touch between hand and arm be as complete as possible. At first massage with very light pressure; gradually develop medium and, finally, strong pressure. Press especially deeply on the left side. Then decrease the pressure, passing gradually through each stage until the pressure is so light that your hand barely touches your belly at all. Take at least five minutes for this massage. This motion follows the curvature of the large intestine.

STEP 2

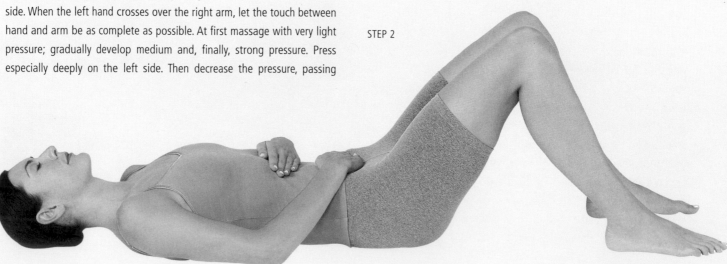

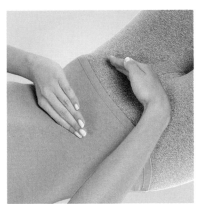

STEP 3

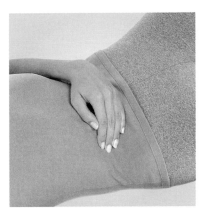

STEP 4

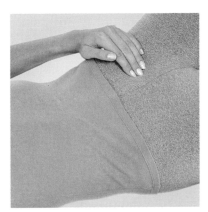

STEP 5

3 Gradually move one hand to the upper border of your belly and the other to the lower border, near the pubic bone. Place the edges of your hands against your body, so the palms face each other. Hold your breath a little, but not very intensely. Slowly push down with the upper hand and up with the lower hand, making your belly into a ball. Be very relaxed in the upper part of your body, especially in your chest and neck. Remember to hold your breath. Exhale slowly, then repeat several times. **4** Place your left hand on your belly, with the fingers pointing to the right. Push your belly out a little and keep it there, breathing gently through nose and mouth. With your hand in place, develop a slow circular movement with the edge of your hand and the tips of your fingers, pressing deeply into your belly, especially on the left side. Continue for several minutes creating a steady rhythm that is linked to the breath. **5** Now in any way that feels appropriate to you, continue to massage the superficial muscles of your belly area. Massage up on the right side of your belly, across the area under the ribs to the left, and down on the left side, following the path of the large intestine. Then massage more deeply, gently kneading all of your internal organs and tissues, starting under the ribs and working down into the pelvic area. Again, work down on the left side and up on the right. When you find a tense place, spend more time there. Breathe easily, and let the breath soften and melt the edges of your tension. When you feel ready to stop, repeat the first stroke in this section — simultaneous circling movements with both hands — to create a natural conclusion. Then lie quietly for a few minutes, breathing gently through both nose and mouth. You can do the belly massage even when it is not convenient for you to lie down. To do it in a sitting position, support your lower back with one hand and rub the belly with the other hand. When you rub in circles, be sure to rub up on the right and down on the left.

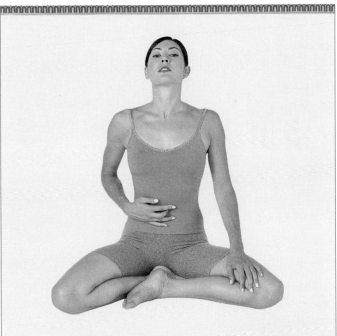

You can also do the following massage in a sitting position: strongly press the navel (there is a pressure point there) with the middle finger of one hand while arching your spine and neck backward. Do not let your head go all the way back. Rest the other hand on your knee. Hold for a minute, breathing gently through nose and mouth. Then slowly straighten your spine while gradually decreasing the pressure. Explore the feelings generated by the massage.

MASSAGE FOR THE ARMS

Massaging the arms improves both breathing and circulation so that the two systems become rhythmic and balanced. In addition, muscles throughout the body are strengthened, and a fresh, pure quality is stimulated within the subtle energies.

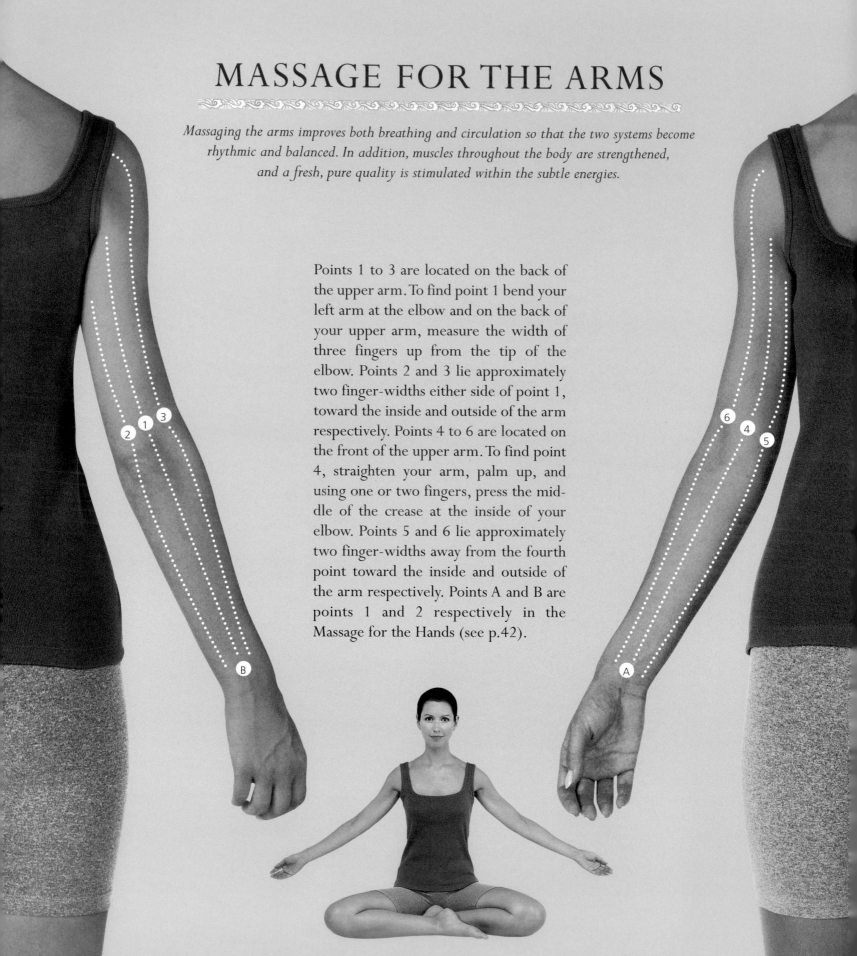

Points 1 to 3 are located on the back of the upper arm. To find point 1 bend your left arm at the elbow and on the back of your upper arm, measure the width of three fingers up from the tip of the elbow. Points 2 and 3 lie approximately two finger-widths either side of point 1, toward the inside and outside of the arm respectively. Points 4 to 6 are located on the front of the upper arm. To find point 4, straighten your arm, palm up, and using one or two fingers, press the middle of the crease at the inside of your elbow. Points 5 and 6 lie approximately two finger-widths away from the fourth point toward the inside and outside of the arm respectively. Points A and B are points 1 and 2 respectively in the Massage for the Hands (see p.42).

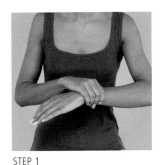

STEP 1

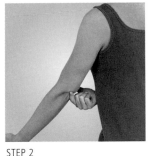

STEP 2

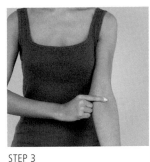

STEP 3

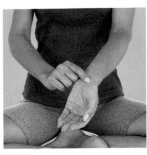

STEP 4

1 Grasp your left wrist with the right hand so that the thumb and middle finger meet at the inside of your wrist. Slowly turn your right hand in one direction until you have made as complete a ring as possible. Massage firmly, squeezing and pressing the arm as you turn your hand. Then shift your hand up your arm one hand-width, and turn your hand in the other direction to make the second ring. By the fourth ring you will be up to or a little beyond the elbow. **2** Press strongly on point 1 with your right forefinger. Straighten your neck as you press. Then slowly stretch out your left arm in front of you, palm up, and continue to press and manipulate this point. Take time to experience what you feel. Then, as if drawing a straight line from this point, slowly rub and press at intervals down the length of

the back of the forearm to point B on the back of the wrist and then back up again. Spend more time working on painful or sensitive spots. You may eventually be able to locate specific nerves in your arm. Repeat this massage with first point 2 and then point 3, working down the back of the forearm in parallel lines from the points to the back of the wrist. **3** Perform this action with points 4 to 6 on the front of the forearm. Begin by pressing point 4 very strongly. Then slowly, rubbing and pressing at intervals, trace a line down to point A on the inside crease of your wrist. Pay special attention to this point. Then work slowly back up to the fourth point. Repeat this action with points 5 and 6. In each case press fairly strongly, allowing the sensations you feel to expand. You will probably find

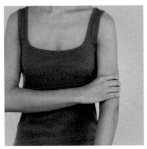

STEP 5

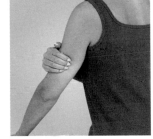

STEP 6

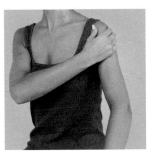

STEP 7

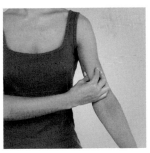

STEP 8

that point 6 is the most sensitive of the three. Rubbing here may release sensations in your neck, heart area and possibly, your intestines. Throughout the massage breathe gently and easily through nose and mouth. **4** Having worked down the forearm from the sixth point, continue a little further beyond the wrist-crease to a special place next to the bone. Press there with your fingers, one at a time, keeping your arm almost straight. Then slowly massage back up to the sixth point, being especially aware of sensations in your heart area. Perform the complete forearm massage on both arms. **5** Following the technique in step 1, massage your upper arm in rings from elbow to shoulder. **6** Massage from each of the three pressure points on the back of the arm up to the top of the shoulder

and down again to the elbow. Do the same for the three pressure points on the front of the arm. Perform this upper arm massage on both arms. **7** Gently massage the deltoid muscle over the shoulder cap, and the biceps muscle on the front of the upper arm until they have no knots or sore areas in them. These muscles both tend to become overdeveloped in men. There should be a continuous flow from one muscle to the next, although each individual muscle should be able to move alone. **8** Rest your hand on your knee, and straighten your arm as you gently massage the biceps with the other hand. Straightening the arm will help to increase the length and freedom of the biceps. Be sure to do the complete upper arm-massage on both arms.

MASSAGE FOR THE BACK

Massaging the back helps to release feelings of joy and love, and gives life and strength to all the senses. The general massages (steps 1 to 5) and the backward-roll massage (steps 6 to 8) shown here relieve muscular tension along the length of the spine, releasing sensations of well-being and joy. Nurture yourself with these feelings; let them touch your heart. As you do these massages, move so gently that your body loses a sense of definite form and you become one with the feeling of joy as it spreads throughout your body. This sensation can become so large and full that it extends beyond your body, and the boundaries between you and the world around you dissolve.

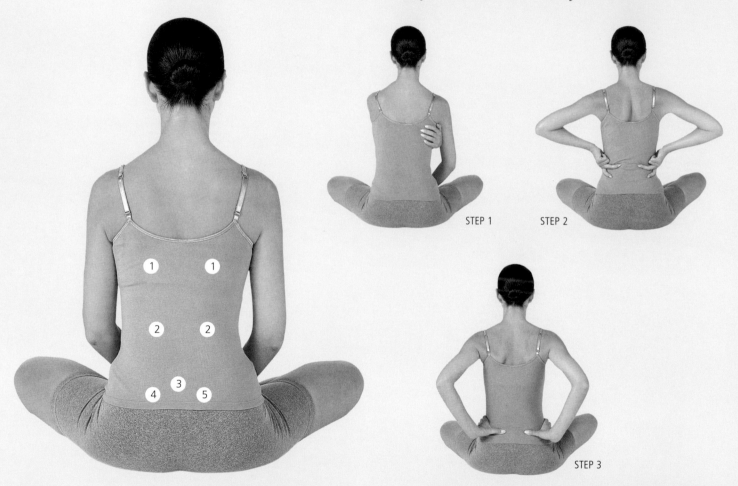

STEP 1   STEP 2

STEP 3

1 Working on first one side of your back and then the other, massage the sides of your chest, in the armpits, and around your torso toward the centre of your back. There are large muscles in this area, so take your time and massage them thoroughly. Then work around and on top of each shoulder blade in turn. Press points 1 (located just above the lower curve of the shoulder blades) with your middle fingers, either at the same time or separately, slowly increasing and decreasing the pressure. **2** Points 2 are located on the muscle at about the level of the kidneys, and are exactly opposite chest points 5 (see p.55). Press points 2 with your middle

fingers, gradually developing strong pressure. Release slowly. Then use one middle finger to press one back point, and the other to press the corresponding chest point. Then do the other pair of points. **3** Use your thumbs to press the points on the sacrum (first point 3, then points 4 and 5 simultaneously), gradually increasing and decreasing the pressure. Then, using your thumbs wherever possible (and your middle fingers when your thumbs cannot reach) strongly press the pairs of points (not shown) between each of the vertebrae, working from the base of the spine all the way up to the base of the skull.

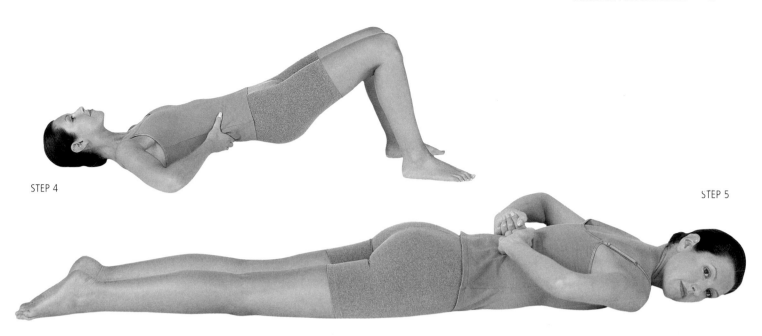

STEP 4

STEP 5

❹ Lie on your back on a mat or soft rug. Separate your legs a comfortable distance, bend your knees and place your feet flat on the floor. Lift your pelvis from the floor, shifting your weight toward your shoulders. Using both hands massage around the sides of your body toward your back. ❺ Now lie on your stomach with your head to one side and massage the sides of your body and your back, moving your hands toward the centre of your back – use your knuckles in this area. ❻ The backward-roll massages the upper area of the back where the hands cannot reach. Sit on the floor with your legs a comfortable distance apart, your knees bent and your feet flat on the floor. Hold the top of your left knee with your left hand and the top of your right knee with your right hand.

Without moving your legs, slowly lean backward until your arms become straight and the small of your back is as close as possible to the floor. ❼ Keeping your hands on top of your knees, slowly draw your feet along the floor toward you and roll backward, straightening your legs as they come over your head. Roll forward to return to a sitting position. Make sure that the small of your back touches the floor during the roll. Perform the roll several times. ❽ Roll backward as before but this time keeping your legs bent and remaining on your back. With your arms around your knees, draw them close to your chest and slowly and gently roll from side to side a little, massaging your back as fully as possible.

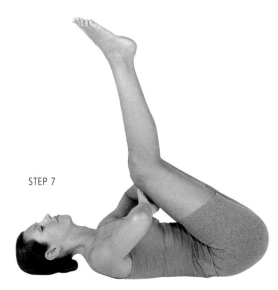

STEP 7

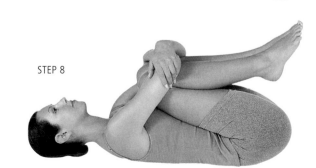

STEP 6

STEP 8

MASSAGE FOR THE LEGS

Massaging the legs is beneficial for everybody: if you do regular vigorous exercise, massaging the legs will smooth the flow of sensation and relieve subtle blockages; if you are relatively inactive, massaging the legs will begin to awaken sleeping energies and encourage their flow.

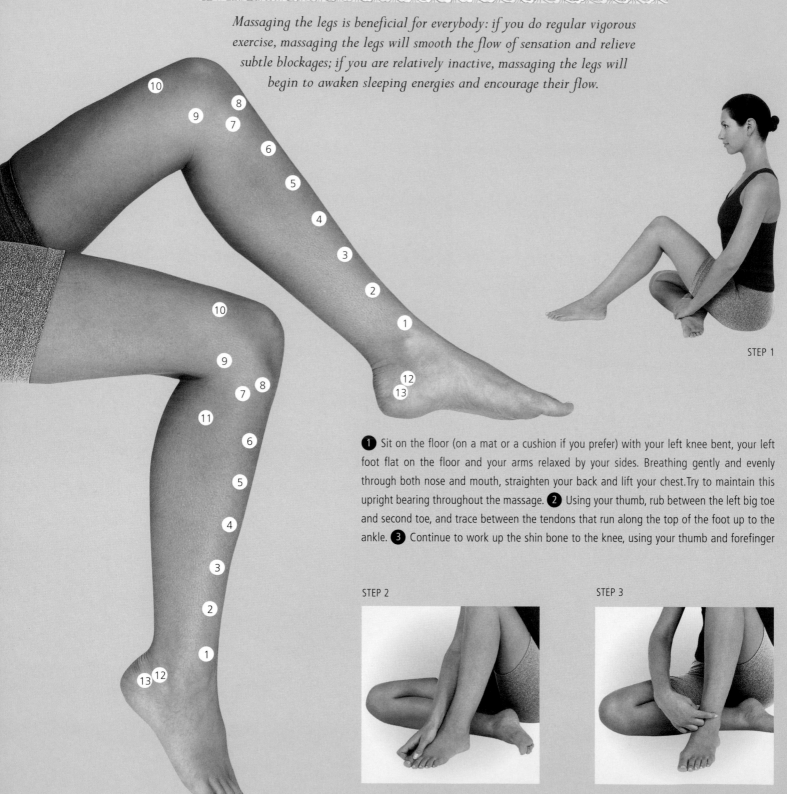

STEP 1

❶ Sit on the floor (on a mat or a cushion if you prefer) with your left knee bent, your left foot flat on the floor and your arms relaxed by your sides. Breathing gently and evenly through both nose and mouth, straighten your back and lift your chest. Try to maintain this upright bearing throughout the massage. ❷ Using your thumb, rub between the left big toe and second toe, and trace between the tendons that run along the top of the foot up to the ankle. ❸ Continue to work up the shin bone to the knee, using your thumb and forefinger

STEP 2

STEP 3

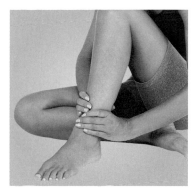

STEP 4

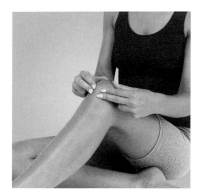

STEP 5

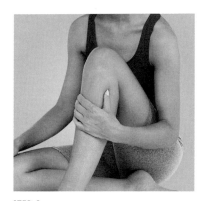

STEP 6

to press points 1 to 6 on either side of the bone. If you find small clusters of tension or pain, rub them in small circles until any knots loosen and dissolve. Breathe gently through both nose and mouth as you rub. Repeat steps 2 and 3 with the right leg. ❹ With both hands grasp your left leg just above the ankle, one hand above the other, thumbs at the back of the leg. Simultaneously twist and press both hands right, then left, as you work up the shin to the kneecap. Hold your leg firmly as you twist, keeping the contact between hands and leg as full as possible. Change the

position of your hands so that the thumbs are on the front of the shin and repeat the leg twist. ❺ Use your fingertips to massage around the kneecap, down the sides of the knee and behind the knee. Then with your thumbs, press the four sets of points (points 7 to 10) that are located on and around the knee. If you do not find these points initially, do not give up; you will find them when you go deeper into your feelings and allow them to guide you. Breathe evenly through both your nose and mouth as you explore with your fingers. When you find a point, experiment with

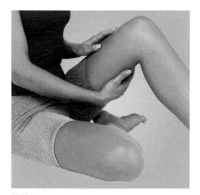

STEP 7

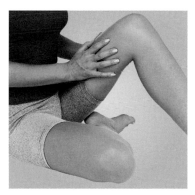

STEP 8

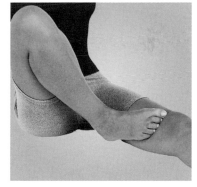

STEP 9

degrees of pressure. ❻ With your thumbs press strongly on point 11, which is approximately five and a half inches (13.7cm) down from the top of the kneecap on the outside of the leg. Release the pressure slowly. ❼ To massage the thigh muscles, place one hand on the back and one hand on the front of the thigh. Moving the hands in first the same direction and then in opposite directions, rub along the thighs in large, sweeping movements, pressing as strongly as you can. Ensure your whole palm is in contact with your leg as you rub. ❽ Then place one hand on the inside and one hand on the outside of the thigh and continue the movements. Explore for any knots or painful spots by tracing the muscles up from the knee area

with your fingers. If you find any tense places, rub these areas with four fingers, using a circular motion. Pay special attention to the places where the thigh muscles join the hip and knee. Now reverse the position of your legs and repeat steps 4 to 8 on the right leg. ❾ Sit with your legs outstretched in front of you and lightly place your palms flat on the floor near your hips. Relax your legs as much as possible. Bend your right knee and place the pad of the foot high up on the left leg, near the groin. Use the right leg and foot to massage the left leg, curling around it and moving up and down its entire length. Continue for several minutes. Then change the position of the legs and massage the left leg with the right.

MASSAGE FOR THE HIPS

Massaging the hip helps to stimulate energies that become blocked from lack of exercise and then spreads these healing and invigorating feelings throughout the whole system.

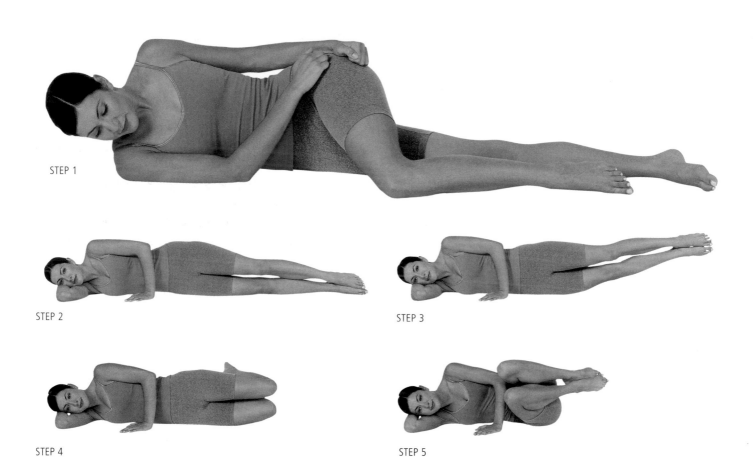

STEP 1

STEP 2

STEP 3

STEP 4

STEP 5

1 Lie down on your right side with your right leg straight, left leg bent over in front of the right. Beginning at the waist, use both hands to massage down the left hip and buttock toward the leg. Try massaging with your fists – small circular movements with the knuckles will help to loosen tension. If you discover any sensitive areas, massage these thoroughly, merging the breath with your sensations and opening the feeling of relaxation as wide as you can. If you do not feel much sensation at first, simply continue to bring your breath and your awareness into the massage and sensation will awaken within you. **2** Tuck one arm under your head as a pillow, and place the other hand flat on the floor near your chest. Straighten your legs and rest your left leg on top of your right. **3** Slowly lift both legs about six inches (15cm) above the ground. **4** Without lowering your legs, bend your knees, pressing your calves as close to your thighs as you can. **5** After holding position 4 briefly, bring your knees in close to your chest. Notice the pressure of your right hip against the floor. Now slowly straighten your legs, lower them to the floor and rest. Repeat slowly two times. As you do so, explore the feelings generated by the massage. Feel the flow of energy from your hip to your lower body and then your upper body. Concentrate on the sensations in the rest of your body, rather than in your hip. Now roll onto your left side and repeat the whole massage on the right side.

MASSAGE FOR THE FEET

*Like massaging the hands, massaging the feet can help to tune and vitalize the whole body. The massage for
the feet comprises two parts: a more general massage (steps 1 to 5) and a points massage (steps 6 to 17). Perform the
entire foot massage twice, the second time a little more slowly. If there are points at which pressure produces a
change in feeling, continue to apply pressure and try to explore the feeling, expanding it as much as possible.
If the massage uncovers a sore spot, massage it gently without lingering over it.*

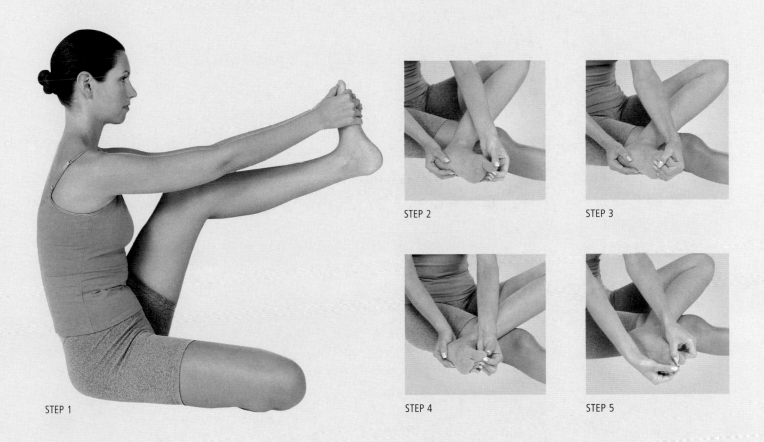

STEP 1

STEP 2

STEP 3

STEP 4

STEP 5

❶ Sit with your legs loosely crossed, the left leg outside the right. Lift
your left knee, interlace your fingers and use them to cradle the ball of your
left foot. Push your foot against your hands, straightening the leg in front
of you as much as possible. Feel the stretch in your leg and the ball of your
foot, and hold briefly. Then slowly lower your leg to the floor. Repeat for
the right leg and foot. ❷ Straighten your right leg and cross the left leg
over the right, resting the left shin on the right thigh. Support the foot with
your right hand on the heel and grasp the toes in your left hand. Vigorously
rotate all the toes together, first in one direction and then in the other. ❸
Extend the circles so that you are rotating the ball of the foot as well as
the toes. The whole upper part of the foot can participate in these circles.
Vary the rhythm, rotating both slowly and quickly. ❹ Still grasping the
toes with the left hand, bend them back and forth several times. Then
extend the motion so the ball of the foot, as well as the toes, bends back
and forth. The foot is very relaxed during this movement. ❺ Begin to massage the toes of the left foot, using the fingers of both hands. Apply ▶

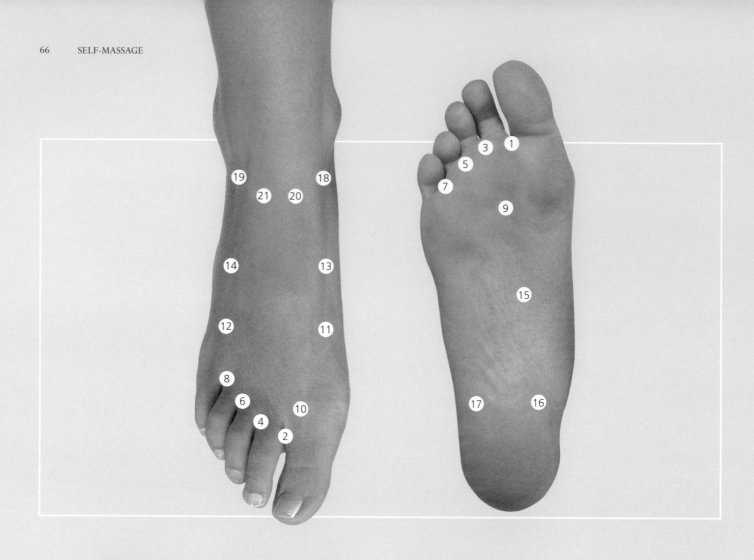

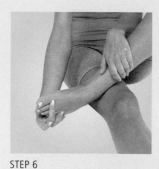

STEP 6

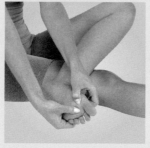

STEP 7

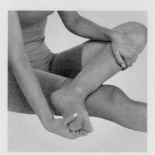

STEP 8

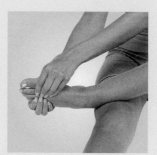

STEP 9

pressure to the pads of the toes. Then massage each toe, one at a time, from the base of the toe to the pad, ensuring that you massage the sides as well as the front and back of each toe. Use direct pressure as well as rotating motions and pull gently on each toe to stretch it. **6** Massage the areas where the toes join the sole, using the thumb or knuckle. With your thumb on the sole and your middle finger on the top of the foot, press points 1 to 8 – the four pairs of points between the bones of the toes. **7** Using the thumbs of both hands, strongly probe each of the toe joints on the ball of the foot. Press deeply between the pads of the ball of the foot. When you find a sensitive place, spend a little longer massaging the area

in order to become acquainted with it – you may find that this releases certain memories. **8** Pay particular attention to point 9, located on the pad of the foot, immediately behind the bulge of the big toe. Use medium to strong pressure on this point, releasing the pressure very slowly. With your thumb on point 9, place your forefinger on point 10 on the top of the foot and massage these two points simultaneously. **9** With your thumbs on the ball of your foot, use your fingers to press the top of the foot, above the ball. Then move the thumbs to the instep and massage the rest of the top of the foot using a rotating pressure, paying particular attention to points 11,12, 13 and 14. **10** Use the knuckles and the fist of the right

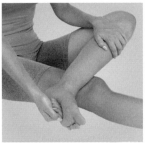
STEP 10

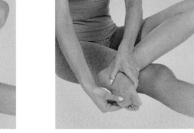
STEP 11

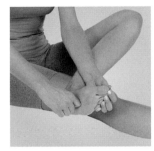
STEP 12

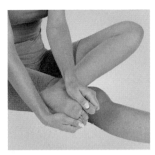
STEP 13

hand to exert pressure everywhere on the sole of the foot, including point 15, in the middle of the sole. **11** Using your thumbs stroke the length of the sole diagonally, starting just in front of the heel on the inside of the foot. Alternate your thumbs, creating a continuous sweeping rhythm. It is important not to break the contact between hand and foot during this part of the massage. Then stroke diagonally from the side of the foot, near the heel, to the ball of the big toe. You may experience different feeling-tones, some of them slightly painful. Breathe into the pain and let it deepen into a nurturing sensation as you exhale. Stroke very slowly, sensing fully, with your belly relaxed. Allow the breath and the stroke to unite with sensation.

12 Arch the toes back with your left hand and jut the heel forward. A valley will form in the middle of the sole when you do this. Using the knuckles or fist of your right hand, press firmly all the points along this valley. The tendon here may feel very tight and sore. You may experience a sudden surge of energy or a rush of warmth around your heart as you press. Explore sensitively, bringing your awareness into whatever you feel. **13** Grasp one side of the ball of the foot with the left hand and the other side with the right hand. Pull your hands apart and slightly away from you as if you are trying to make the sole convex. Maximize the contact between your hands and feet as you pull. Then pull the sides of the feet toward you as if

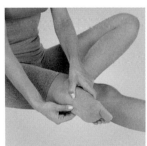

STEP 14

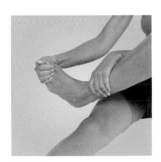
STEP 15

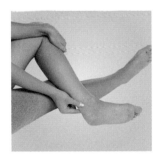
STEP 16

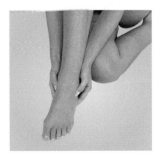
STEP 17

trying to make the sole concave. **14** Pinch and probe all the areas around the heel, pressing points 16 and 17 strongly. **15** Grasp the toes of the left foot with your right hand and rest your left hand on the left leg just above the ankle. With your foot relaxed, slowly rotate the ankle in a circle, first in one direction, and then in the other. Let your hand do the work; your foot should be completely relaxed. If you feel a tight place, explore it by moving more slowly and breathing gently. Allow any tensions throughout your body to dissolve. Continue the rotations for several minutes, until they become smooth and easy. **16** Vigorously pinch and rub the Achilles tendon at the back of the foot. **17** Apply pressure to all points on and

around the ankle, including points 18 to 21, as well as points 12 and 13 from the Massage for the Legs (see p.62), which are located in the hollow just below the ankle bones. Now position your foot so that you can massage the top of it comfortably. Rub between the toes and trace between the tendons, working up to the ankle. Include the sides of the foot in your massage. To finish try this simple test. Stand up, resting your weight equally on each foot. How do the two feet relate to the ground? Do you notice any differences? Does one foot feel light, the other heavy? Does there appear to be an energetic quality in one foot that contrasts with a sense of dullness in the other? Now repeat the foot massage on the right foot.

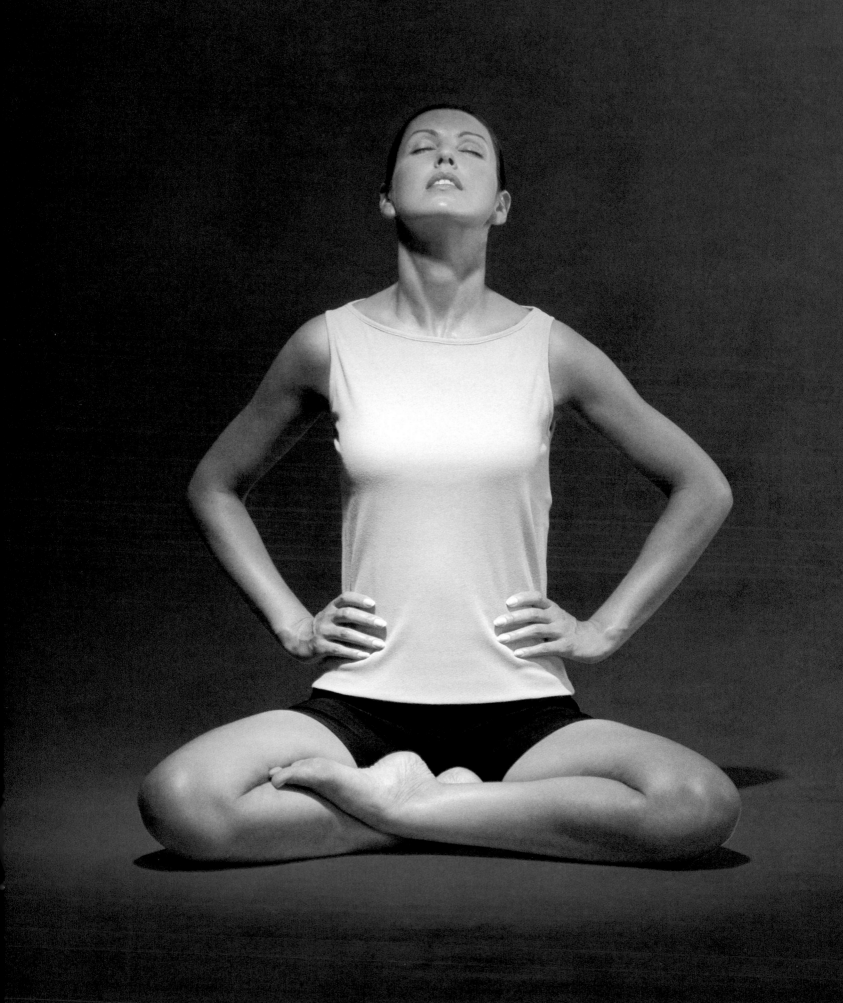

CHAPTER FOUR

GENTLE MOVEMENT

*"Once you have tasted inner relaxation,
your body will be your truest guide."*

Exercise that is genuine and pure, uniting body and mind, truly revitalizes our energies and sustains us in our daily lives. This chapter introduces us to such exercise with a selection of gentle movement exercises, which activate the first stage of the Kum Nye internal "energy massage". During these exercises we are encouraged to bring breath and awareness to our bodies and senses as we move slowly in certain ways. This gives us the opportunity to contact the feelings and sensations that interconnect the mind, body and senses. Once this is achieved we can release and expand these feelings in order to transform them into healing, invigorating energies. The chapter also shows how we can combine these gentle movement exercises with the breathing exercises and self-massages to form a basic practice for beginners.

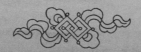

GUIDING PRACTICE

"Once the flow of feeling is stimulated, each exercise becomes an opportunity to explore the ease that characterizes the harmonious relationship between body, breath, senses, mind and environment."

The gentle movement exercises in this chapter provide the foundation for all the Kum Nye movement exercises, activating the processes of relaxation that are developed further in later exercises. As a result they should form the basis of your movement practice during the first four to six months.

The exercises

Try to practise Kum Nye as regularly as you can. Forty-five minutes a day is a good length of time to practise these exercises, although as little as twenty minutes will bring long-term results. Try not to worry if you miss a day or so; you will not lose ground. Simply encourage yourself and continue to practise when you can – even doing an exercise for five or ten minutes on a break from work can have a beneficial effect.

If possible, spend fifteen to twenty minutes working on every exercise, performing each one three or nine times and spending at least two or three minutes on every repetition. (Each repetition is an opportunity to explore the feelings activated by the movement more fully, a chance to bring body, mind and senses together.) Afterwards sit quietly for five to ten minutes. As you progress you may want to practise for longer periods of time. If you feel strong emotions during an exercise, sit quietly and relax for a moment before continuing. If you feel unwell, take care not to do too much.

Level one

Spend the first two or three months working with the exercises from level one. To start with, choose two or three exercises that appeal to you and practise each one daily for about fifteen minutes each (you may want to experiment with a number of the exercises to find out which ones suit you best). After a few weeks, swap these for two or three of the other exercises and practise these every day for a few weeks.

The exercises in this group release tension in the spine and upper body – particularly the shoulders, neck and head. During stretching exercises be careful not stretch too much or too quickly as this may strain muscles and cause a heavy, inert state of mind. Instead ease gently into stretches, breathing evenly through both nose and mouth, and developing a quality of lightness throughout your body. This distributes feeling and energy evenly throughout the body, with the result that you begin to feel more in your heart.

These simple exercises help us to develop the abundance of our inner resources. Even if nothing appears to be happening while you do an exercise, a change will gradually be occurring in the quality of your daily life. Every aspect of your experience will seem clearer and more vital as your senses begin to open and their perceptions become more substantial, full and alive.

Level two

After a few months, swap one or two exercises at a time from level two into your movement practice, spending a few weeks working with each before moving onto any others. At this point in your practice, you have already begun to touch and develop the feelings and sensations that relax and nurture you. The exercises in level two will help you to deepen these experiences further, introducing new feeling-tones, which can be expanded and enriched.

Extending your practice

After spending a few months on these exercises, you may feel ready to look at some of the exercises in chapters five and six. The level one and two exercises in these chapters will extend the process of relaxation that you have already begun; the level three exercises will give you an idea of how Kum Nye can be developed further.

POINTS FOR PRACTICE

The following points are applicable to all of the movement exercises, from the most basic level one exercises in this chapter, to the most advanced level three exercises in chapter six. Bear them in mind when working through each exercise — they will help you to gain maximum benefit from your practice.

When selecting exercises and developing sequences, allow your body to guide you. If you are unused to exercising, be gentle with yourself. Do not try to do too much: remember it is the quality of the movement that is most important. If you have any injuries, use your judgment when choosing exercises: pay attention to any warnings given in the exercise introductions, and in the exercises that you select, move very gently with awareness of your body. If you are pregnant or have undergone an operation in the last three or four months, work on the gentler exercises on pp. 76, 79, 81 and 86–7.

Try not to rush your practice. Coverage and speed are not important. Stay with each exercise until it opens up your senses and you become aware of the feelings and sensations in your body. Within each exercise move very slowly and smoothly – this will allow you to be sensitive to variations in your feelings and help you to develop the quality of your practice. Throughout each exercise breathe evenly through both nose and mouth, so that your energies are constantly balanced.

Pay attention to the particular flavours of the feelings that arise during each exercise. Remember not to name or label the feeling-tones of your experience; simply be aware of their qualities – their texture and weight, their sense of time. Do not worry if your feelings or sensations do not match the feelings or sensations mentioned in the exercise descriptions; these descriptions are only indications of what you might feel.

Continue to explore your feelings in a sensitive way during the sitting period of each exercise. The sitting posture (see p.28) that is adopted during this period encourages an even flow of feeling throughout your body. If you wish, try sitting for a few minutes before your practice. This will help you to develop a meditative awareness as you centre your focus in your body. At the end of your practice incorporate Kum Nye into your next activity by continuing to expand your feelings, whether you are eating, walking or simply observing the world around you. As relaxation comes to inform every experience, your whole life will become part of an expanding meditation.

You may find that some of the exercises have an immediate effect, some affect you gradually and some do not appear to affect you at all. If, after several practice sessions, an exercise does not appear to be generating much feeling or energy, you could be holding some tension that is blocking the flow of sensation. You may be holding a particular position too rigidly. Try moving a little within the position to relax any tension and release a different quality of energy. If the exercise continues to have little effect, leave it for a while. You may find it effective when you return to it at a later date.

There may be times when you find that you are unable to touch your feelings during an exercise. This can indicate that your body and mind are too excited or tense to communicate effectively with each other: your mind may be so full of thoughts and images that you are unable to sense your feelings clearly; you may be too upset to breathe in the even and gentle way that awakens nurturing feelings. To calm and relax you in preparation for your practice, try sitting quietly for a few minutes, concentrating lightly on your breathing.

LOOSENING UP

This exercise relaxes the upper back, especially the muscles of the shoulder blades. It also relaxes the hips.
At the end sit quietly in the sitting posture for five to ten minutes, distributing the sensations
awakened by the exercise to your whole body, and beyond, to the surrounding universe.

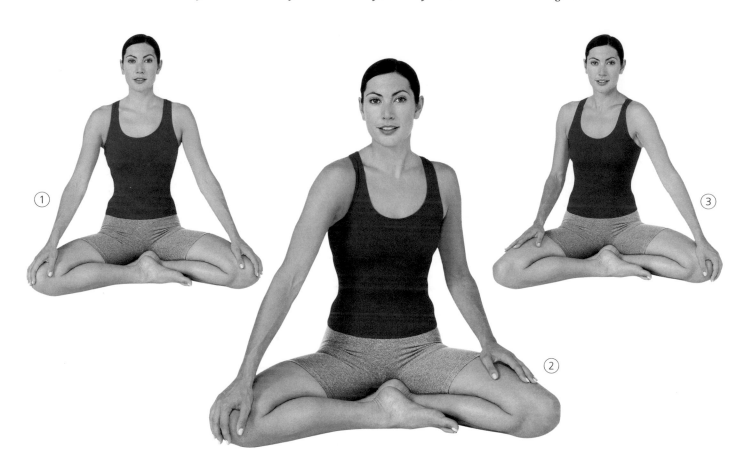

1 Sit cross-legged on a mat or cushion with your hands on your knees and your arms straight.

2 Keeping your chest facing forward and breathing easily through both nose and mouth, simultaneously move your right shoulder forward as far as possible and your left shoulder back as far as possible. Keep your right arm straight and let the left elbow bend. Take about 15 seconds for this movement. The shoulders should move independently of the head. This may feel a little strange at first.

3 Slowly move your left shoulder forward as your right shoulder moves back, straightening your left arm and allowing your right elbow to bend. Move very slowly, sensing the feelings awakened in your body. Feel the stretch in your back and neck at the end of the movement; you may feel sensations of warmth there.

Do the complete movement 3 or 9 times.

TOUCHING FEELING

This exercise releases tension in the neck and shoulders. At the end sit in the sitting posture for five to ten minutes, expanding your sensations and feelings.

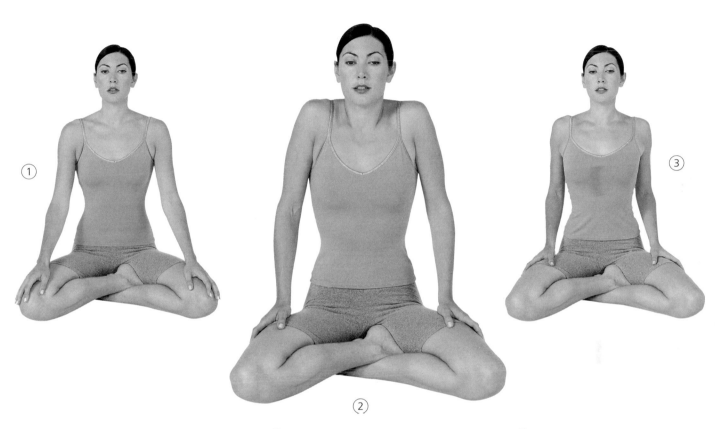

1 Sit cross-legged on a mat or cushion with your hands on your knees. Relax your belly.

This exercise can also be done standing. When attempting this variation allow your arms to hang relaxed and close to your body as you rotate your shoulders in the shoulder joints.

2 Inhale and slowly lift your shoulders as high as possible, allowing the position of your hands to shift as needed. When you think your shoulders are as high as they can go, relax while still holding them up, and you may find that they can be raised a little more. Let your neck settle down between your shoulders. Now hold your breath a little and lightly imagine the back of your neck to be fresh and warm like that of a happy baby.

3 Very slowly exhale, as you do so rotating your shoulders back and down, feeling the sensations in the back of your neck and spine. Keep your belly relaxed. Let your hands and arms be very relaxed – you may feel sensations of warmth and softness there.

Slowly continue to rotate your shoulders forward, up, back and down 3 or 9 times, spending at least 1 minute on each rotation. Then find a place in the movement where you can comfortably change direction and make 3 or 9 rotations the other way.

LIGHTENING THOUGHTS

This exercise relieves tension in the neck, head and shoulders, and lightens the fixed quality of thoughts and images. Avoid this exercise if you are pregnant or have had any kind of neck injury, and perform it particularly slowly if your neck muscles are tight. At the end sit in the sitting posture for ten minutes, expanding your feelings and energy.

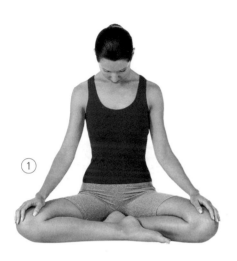
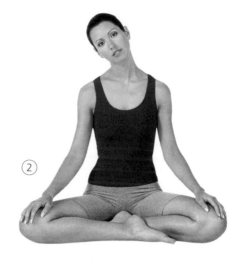
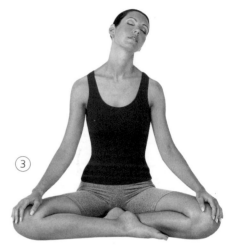

① Sit cross-legged on a mat or cushion with your hands on your knees. With your mouth slightly open, breathing gently, very slowly lower your chin toward your chest. Then very slowly lift your chin until it points toward the ceiling. Repeat this very slow lifting and lowering of the chin several times.

② Very slowly move your head so that your right ear moves in the direction of your right shoulder, and then so your left ear moves in the direction of your left shoulder. Repeat several times.

Throughout the exercise breathe very slowly and evenly through both nose and mouth. If the breathing is too fast or uneven, this exercise can produce effects such as nausea or disorientation.

③ Close your eyes and slowly rotate your head clockwise. Relax your shoulders. Make the circle as large as possible without straining. At tight or painful places, move your head back and forth very slowly, allowing the muscles to loosen. You may discern a thought related to the tightness. Slow the rotation until the movement is barely perceptible. Be aware of your whole body, even your toes and fingertips.

Do the clockwise rotation 3 or 9 times. Then change direction, and begin 3 or 9 counterclockwise rotations. On the last rotation, move your head more and more slowly until it finally stops.

During the rotation, concentrate loosely on the juncture of your skull and spine, under the occiput (the back part of the head). You may feel a special energy there, almost a sense of home. Deepen this feeling and expand it as much as you can. Use the spine as a channel for this feeling, distributing it throughout your body. Expand the feeling so that it extends beyond your body, on and on.

REVITALIZING ENERGY

Perform this exercise whenever you feel in need of an energy boost, or some mental or physical refreshment. At the end of the exercise, sit in the sitting posture for five to ten minutes, breathing gently and amplifying your sensations until they fill the space around you.

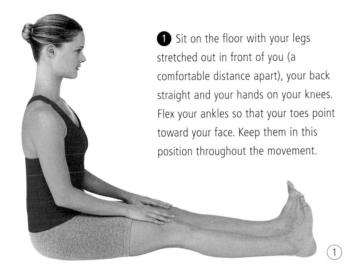

1 Sit on the floor with your legs stretched out in front of you (a comfortable distance apart), your back straight and your hands on your knees. Flex your ankles so that your toes point toward your face. Keep them in this position throughout the movement.

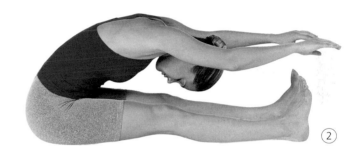

2 Slowly lift your arms to shoulder-height in front of you, palms down. Slowly reach toward your toes, lowering your head between your arms.

Remember to breathe gently and evenly through both nose and mouth throughout the movement.

3 Very slowly draw back, keeping your arms stretched out in front of you and letting your head come up, until you are leaning back a little.

Repeat the forward and backward movements once more, reaching very slowly toward your toes and drawing back even more slowly, expanding the sensations that arise. Feel the qualities of space and time. Do the whole movement 3 or 9 times.

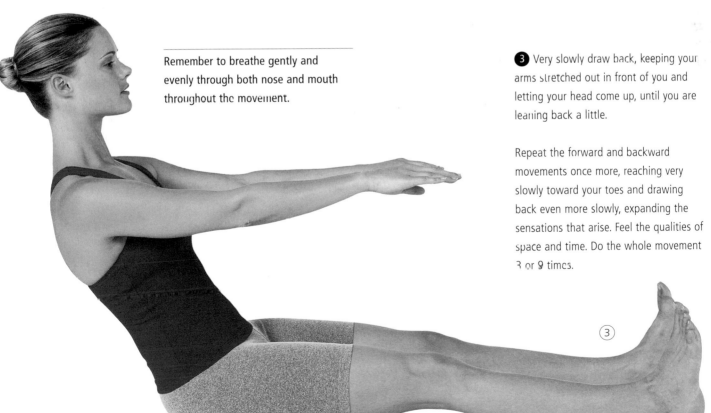

HAND MAGIC

This exercise is a wonderful reminder that the body not only exists, but that it can also give energy and ease to the mind. At the end of the exercise, gradually slow the movement of your hands, allowing them to come to rest in your lap — the back of one hand held in the palm of the other, your head bent slightly forward. Relax your shoulders. Imagine your hands encircling the energy as you bring it to rest. Sit for five to ten minutes, expanding the sensations in your body.

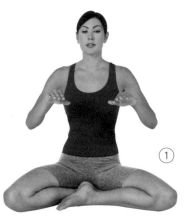

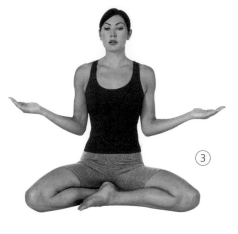

❶ Sit cross-legged, hands on knees. Slowly lift your hands to chest-level in front of you, keeping your elbows bent, palms down. Relax your elbows and move them away from your body slightly. Breathing softly and evenly through both nose and mouth, slowly move your hands up and down from the wrists until you feel heat beneath your hands. Eyes half-closed, watch the hand motion with your peripheral vision. Relax your shoulders and slow the movement of your hands until you see hardly any movement at all. Do you feel heat in your palms, your chest, at the back of your neck, behind your spinal cord? If you feel no heat, you may be moving too fast. Let your hands hang from your wrists and move very lightly, making the motion so small it becomes barely perceptible. Do you feel anything in your hands? Perhaps heat or a tingling sensation?

❷ Once you feel something in your palms or fingers, keep your hands in front of you and slowly turn the palms up. Press your elbows into your sides and push your chest out slightly. Keeping your palms up, slowly move your hands toward each other until they are almost touching, feeling the sensations of heat and energy.

❸ Just before your hands touch, begin to move them apart, until you have separated them as much as possible. Keep the elbows in the same position throughout. Can you still feel the energy?

Continue this forward and backward movement of the forearms 3 or 9 times. Then, with your palms up and elbows pressed into your sides, move your hands toward and away from each other in a very fast, short, strong, shaking motion. Keep your neck straight, relax your belly and let strength pass from your shoulders into your hands. Continue for 30 seconds to 1 minute.

This exercise is most effective when done after massaging or energizing the hands.

TOUCHING BODY ENERGY

This exercise relieves tension in the back of the neck, the spine and the backs of the legs, and redistributes energy and feeling throughout the body. It is not recommended if you are pregnant or have had any back or neck injuries. At the end of the exercise, sit quietly in the sitting posture for five to ten minutes, expanding the sensations awakened by the movement.

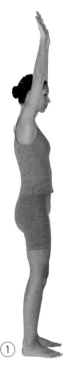

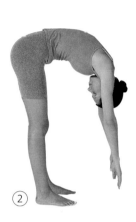

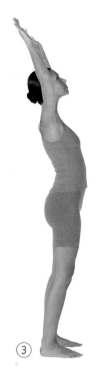

❶ Stand with your feet a comfortable distance apart, your back straight and your body balanced. Breathing softly through both nose and mouth, slowly raise your arms in front of you until they are overhead, with the palms facing forward.

❷ Knees relaxed and straight but not locked, slowly and evenly arch forward from the waist, reaching out slightly with your arms. Your head, torso and arms should move together. Relax your neck muscles and release any tension in your chest, belly and lower energy centres. When your fingers approach the floor, stay down briefly, concentrating lightly on your back. Be very still. Slowly spread your fingers. Exhale fully, releasing tension from your belly so that the flow of energy is not blocked.

❸ Breathing evenly and gently, rise very slowly, keeping your head between your arms. Focus on your throat as you do so — you may feel a sense of opening there. When you reach an upright position, bend backward slightly. Keep your exhalations gentle and allow the front of your body to open, especially your belly, chest and throat.

Slowly straighten your neck and back, bringing your attention to the base of your skull. You may feel warmth there, or a general sense of connection and peace. Again bend forward as before, moving as gently and slowly as possible. Perform the exercise 3 or 9 times.

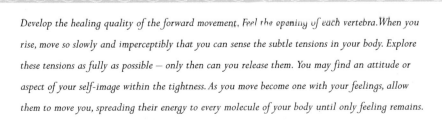

Develop the healing quality of the forward movement. Feel the opening of each vertebra. When you rise, move so slowly and imperceptibly that you can sense the subtle tensions in your body. Explore these tensions as fully as possible — only then can you release them. You may find an attitude or aspect of your self-image within the tightness. As you move become one with your feelings, allow them to move you, spreading their energy to every molecule of your body until only feeling remains.

HEALING BODY AND MIND

This exercise relieves tension in the muscles along the sides of the body. At the end sit in the
sitting posture for five to ten minutes, expanding the feelings stimulated by the exercise.

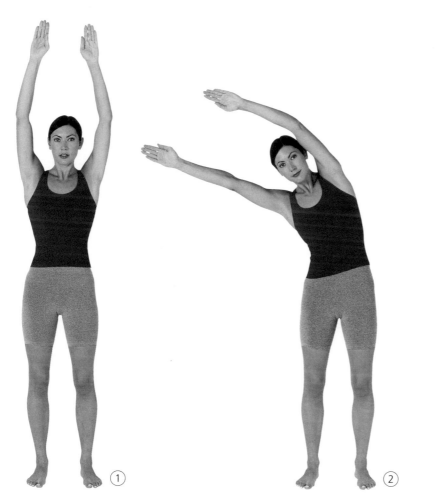

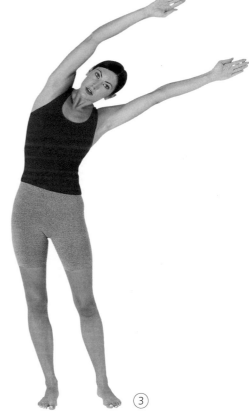

❶ Stand with your body well-balanced, your feet about a foot (30cm) apart, your back straight and your arms relaxed at your sides. Inhale through both nose and mouth and slowly lift your arms in front of you until they are overhead, with the palms facing forward.

❷ While exhaling, slowly bend to the right side, reaching out with your arms and keeping your knees straight but not locked. Let your pelvis move slightly to the left so your weight is balanced on both feet and the curve on both sides of your body is long and graceful. Let your left arm come close to your ear, and your right arm lower a little toward the ground. Keep your mouth slightly open and allow your breath to flow evenly.

❸ While inhaling, slowly return to an upright position and in a continuous motion reach to the opposite side while exhaling. Let your belly be relaxed and empty. Move as slowly as you can, feeling the sensations within your body. Repeat the complete movement 3 or 9 times, relaxing more each time.

This movement can also be done with the palms facing each other.

FLYING

This exercise calms the restless flow of thoughts and generates feeling in the heart centre. To complete the exercise sit in the sitting posture for five minutes or more, continuing to sense the flow of energy, with breath, body and mind as one. As a variation try slowing the movement down, taking two minutes in each direction.

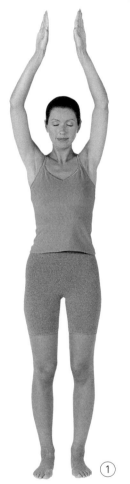

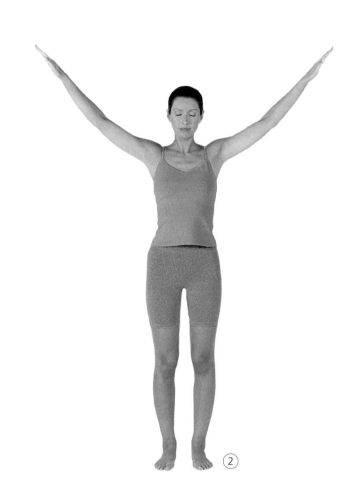

As you move your arms, pay attention to the feeling-tones and the flow of energy through your body. As your arms descend let energy flow into your heart centre; as you raise your arms, direct energy outward through your fingers. You may feel heat and energy surrounding your arms and hands.

❶ Stand well-balanced with your feet about 4 inches (10cm) apart, your back straight and your arms relaxed at your sides. Slowly lift your arms away from your sides until they are directly overhead with the backs of the hands facing each other and the fingers straight. Close your eyes and feel the sensations of energy in your body. Relax your thighs and minimize any backward arching in your spine.

❷ Slowly open your arms, increasing the distance between them in a balanced and equal way. Take 1 full minute to bring them all the way down to your sides.

Take another minute to move your arms up again. When your arms are overhead, stretch up slightly, keeping your legs relaxed. This stretch clears and settles the mind. Do the movement 9 times.

BALANCING BODY AND MIND

This exercise stretches the upper leg and stimulates energy in the sacrum and spine. At the end of the exercise, sit for ten to fifteen minutes, allowing the sensations stimulated by the posture to expand.

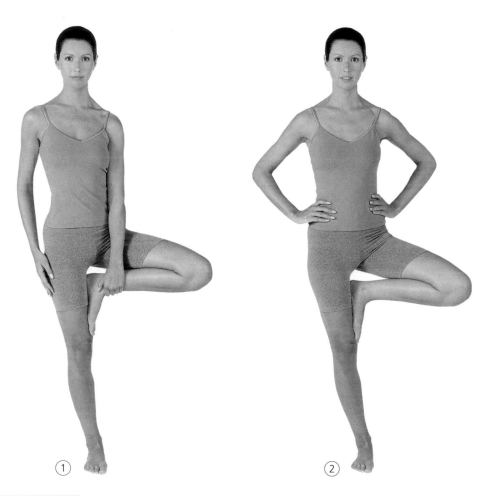

① ②

As you perform this exercise, try to relax and explore the feelings that are awakened within you. With regular practice you will find that different feeling-states produce different feeling-tones — for example, you may find it harder to hold your balance when feeling emotional, or physically tight.

❶ Stand on the floor or ground with your feet a comfortable distance apart and your back straight. Slowly lift your left leg, bending it at the knee. Grasp the inside of the leg near the ankle with your left hand and place the sole of your left foot, toes down, against the inside of your upper right thigh, with the heel near the crotch. Press the heel lightly into your thigh to hold the leg in position.

❷ Move the left knee out to the side, place your hands on your hips, look ahead with soft eyes, and balance. Remain here for 1 to 3 minutes.

Slowly reduce the pressure of your left foot against your right thigh. Now lower your foot to the floor, noting what you feel just before your foot touches the ground. Do the complete movement, first on one side and then the other, 3 times.

BEING AND BODY

This exercise heightens our awareness of the balance between the mind and the body. It is a walking meditation that develops the focused concentration of a seated practice, without the discomfort that can arise during periods of prolonged stillness. You can also practise this exercise walking twice as slowly, covering ten yards (nine metres), back and forth, twice in forty-five minutes.

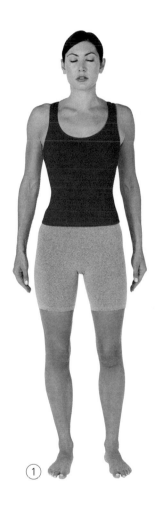
①

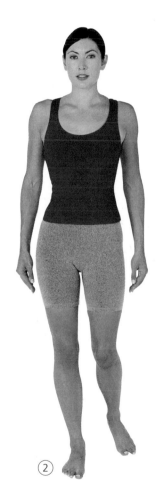
②

2 Now slowly open your eyes, look straight ahead and begin to walk very slowly, taking very small steps – as little as 2 inches (5cm) and not more than 4 inches (10cm). Walk as slowly as you can imagine walking. Then slow down even more. Step very lightly, balancing both sides of your body, your concentration, your breath. Between lifting and stepping there is a kind of silence. Tension in the energy centres, especially in the throat centre, can block this silent quality, so at the moment of lifting your foot from the ground it is important to relax your throat, as well as your belly, knees, shoulders, hands and spine. Relax your awareness, so that your concentration does not become too focused.

Practise this slow walking for 45 minutes, moving so slowly that you cover 10 yards (9m), back and forth, 4 times.

1 Stand well-balanced with your feet a comfortable distance apart, your back straight, and your arms relaxed at your sides. Breathe softly through both nose and mouth. Close your eyes and let tension ebb from your body, especially your chest and throat. Take several minutes to sense how tiny adjustments in muscles and energy affect your balance.

Throughout the exercise give the same emphasis and amount of time to each part of the movement – lifting, moving, stepping. Open your senses in such a way that you do not focus on any particular sense – you should be no more aware of seeing than of hearing. Give as much power to your feelings as to your eyes, ears and thoughts. Feel as much as you think. Give all aspects of your experience equal weight, letting your body and senses operate as a complete whole. As you walk be aware of the mantra OM AH HUM – you do not need to actually pronounce it, simply listen to it inwardly.

CALMING INNER ENERGY

This exercise calms the internal organs and the nervous system and may bring you to a very still place where you have few or no thoughts. If this happens, slow the movement even more, expanding this feeling. When you finish the exercise, sit in the sitting posture for five to ten minutes, continuing to follow and extend the sensations stimulated by the movement.

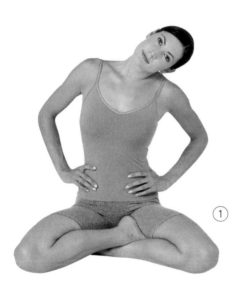

1 Sit cross-legged on a mat or cushion with your back straight and your hands on your hips. Slowly begin to move your upper body in a circle. Bend slowly from the waist to your left, breathing evenly through both your nose and mouth, your head and neck relaxed and hanging.

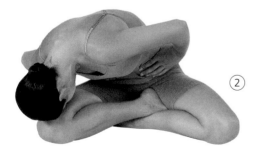

2 Move slowly forward so that your head skims your left knee, passes close to the ground and then skims your right knee.

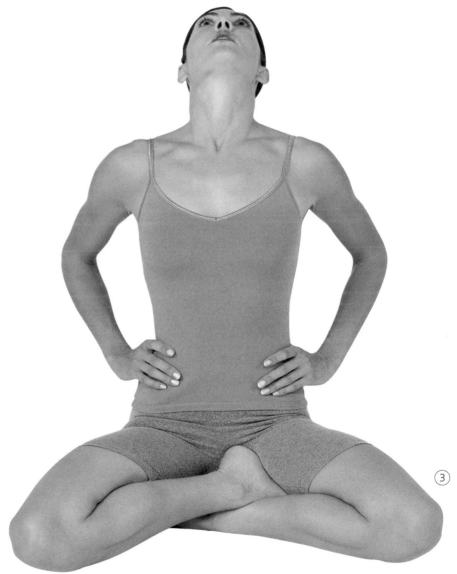

3 Move up on the right side, then arch backward slightly, looking toward the ceiling. Without stopping, continue the circle to the left. Keep your mouth slightly open. Breathe normally during the revolution, except in the forward position, when you should exhale fully. After 9 clockwise rotations, change directions and continue for 9 counterclockwise rotations.

TOUCHING NURTURING FEELING

This exercise stretches the muscles and ligaments between the bones of the upper body, especially the upper spine, and circulates energy to the spine and joints. During the exercise be as relaxed and open as possible — not holding back, not specifically focused on anything. At the end sit in the sitting posture for ten to fifteen minutes, expanding the sensations generated by the holding and releasing of tension.

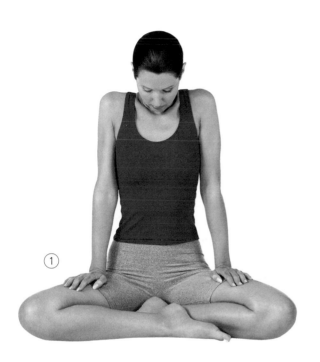

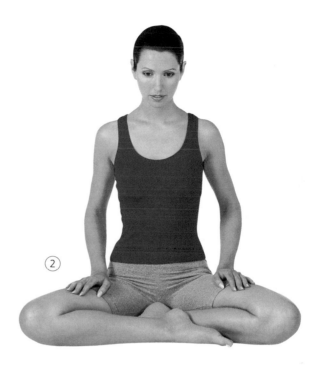

1 Sit comfortably on a mat or cushion in a cross-legged position, knees wide apart and back straight. Place your hands on the tops of your upper thighs, fingers pointing forward. Slowly push your hands against your thighs so that your arms straighten and both shoulders lift as high as possible. Relax your body, and your shoulders may move up a little more. Settle your neck down between your shoulders; your chin will almost touch your chest. Breathe lightly through both nose and mouth, keeping your throat and belly as relaxed as possible. Hold for 3 to 5 minutes, raising energy from the belly area into your chest.

2 After 3 to 5 minutes, very slowly loosen your shoulders a little. Do not rotate your shoulders as they loosen; simply release the tension gradually and allow your shoulders to move downward. Your elbows will bend as your arms relax. Take at least 1 minute for the release. Feel energy flowing down the length of your spine, from the neck to the lower back and sacrum.

Adopt position 1 once more, making your belly a little smaller, and tightening the back of your spine. Breathe slowly through both nose and mouth. If you feel pain, move your shoulders slightly so that energy flows smoothly. Hold this position for 3 to 5 minutes. Then, very slowly relax the tension and feel the deep, sensitive feeling that arises. You may feel warmth in your chest and the back of your neck or a sensation of opening in the chest, throat and head, a feeling of expanding beyond your body.

Perform the entire exercise 3 or 9 times.

When you first do this exercise, the energy will flow down the spine, then forward and up inside your body to the throat, then back down the spine. With practice you will be able to move the energy to all parts of your body.

BODY OF KNOWLEDGE

This exercise relieves eye strain and general tiredness. It also helps to build muscles and to improve the functioning of the joints. If you have had any kind of back or neck injury, or have had an operation within three or four months, move carefully in this exercise and do less than the directions indicate. At the end of the exercise, sit for ten to fifteen minutes, continuing to expand the sensations within and around your body.

❶ Sit cross-legged on a mat or cushion. Place your hands on your knees, fingers pointing toward each other, fingers and thumbs together and elbows pointing out to the sides.

❷ Arch your head forward and down moving your chin toward your chest. Slowly bend forward from the waist, pressing your hands against your knees, pushing your elbows forward. Gently draw in your belly and hold it tightly, breathing evenly through nose and mouth. Each time you exhale let each section of your spine open and expand. When you have bent forward as far as possible, focus lightly on the base of your spine, where you may feel a sense of opening and warmth. Try to expand these feelings. Stay down for 3 to 5 minutes. Just before coming up, change your hand position so the fingers and thumbs point forward. As you come up, press your hands strongly against your legs. The tension may cause shaking; if this occurs notice what you feel.

Very slowly release the tension and sit for 5 minutes, expanding your feelings. Do the movement 3 or 9 times, sitting for 5 minutes after each repetition.

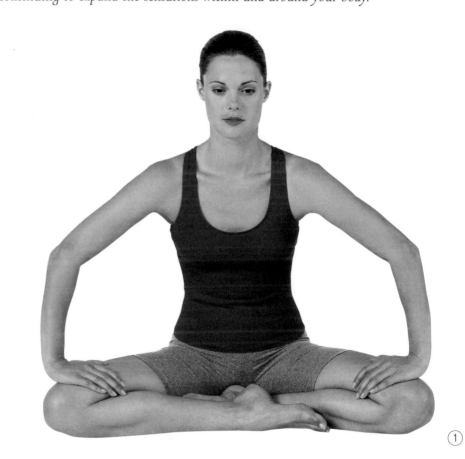

①

②

This variation of the exercise is a little more difficult. At the end sit for five to ten minutes, continuing to expand the sensations at the base of your spine and in your chest and throat, until they are distributed throughout your body and have become part of the space that surrounds you.

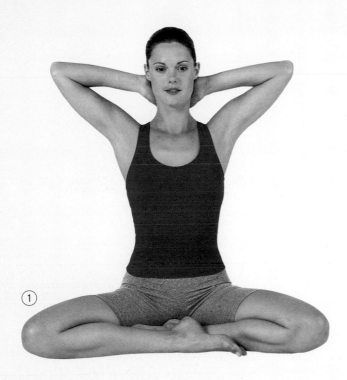

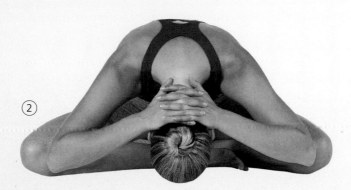

1 Sit on a mat or cushion with your legs loosely crossed. The position of your legs will affect your balance so you may want to experiment with different ways of crossing them until you find the position that permits the most balanced movement. Interlace your fingers and place them on the back of your neck, keeping your elbows out.

2 Slowly push your neck down with your hands so that your chin moves toward your chest. In this position, bend forward slowly from the waist, breathing lightly and evenly through both nose and mouth, with your belly drawn tightly in. As you exhale, let each part of your spine open and expand. When you have bent forward as far as you can without straining, focus lightly on the base of your spine, allowing the sensations there to expand like a halo.

Then, without releasing your hands, come up as slowly as you can. As your spine straightens, hold some strength in the muscles of your chest, as if directing a flow of energy through your chest up into your throat. Then slowly lower your hands to your knees and sit for a few minutes, breathing gently and evenly through both nose and mouth. Perform the exercise 3 or 9 times.

EXPANDING AWARENESS

This exercise expands awareness and concentration, and releases tension in the upper back and shoulders.
Try it after sitting for fifteen to thirty minutes. At the end of the exercise, sit for five to ten minutes,
continuing to expand the sensations of energy both within and outside your body.

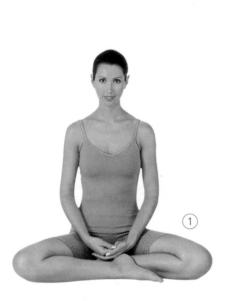

1 Sit cross-legged on a mat or cushion, and place your hands in your lap with the palms up, the right hand held in the left. Loosen your belly and chest, settle your neck down between your shoulders and relax any tension in your spine.

2 Gracefully lift your arms overhead, finishing with the palms facing forward.

3 Imagine a huge ball of energy in front of you. Slowly open your arms and move them down in lateral arcs, as if encircling this ball of energy with your hands. Feel the sensations of energy in your hands and arms.

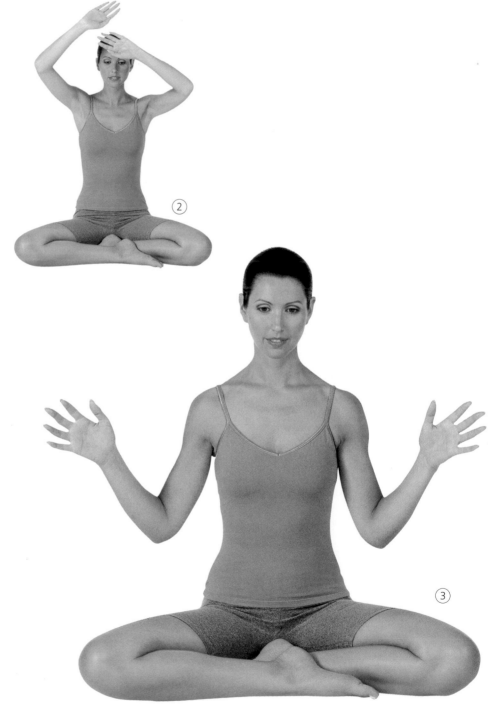

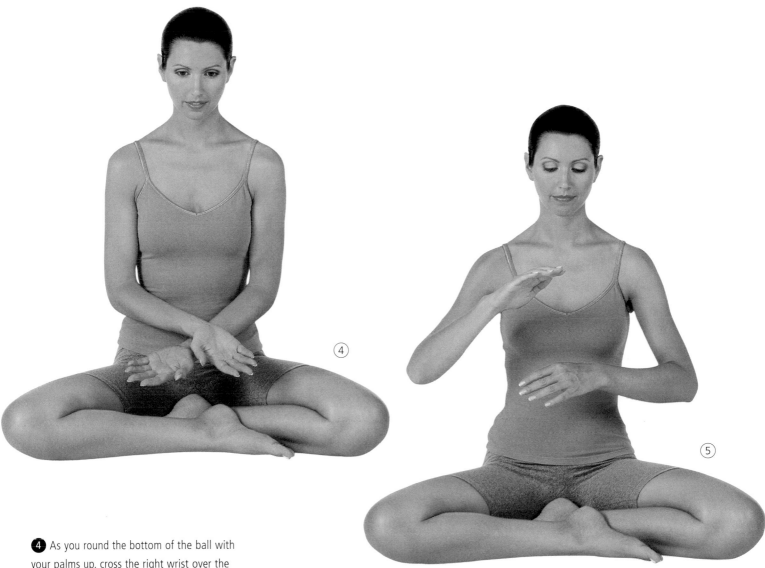

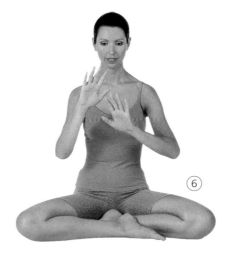

4 As you round the bottom of the ball with your palms up, cross the right wrist over the left without touching them together.

5 In a continuing movement, begin to twist both wrists so that the palms rotate away from you, while simultaneously lifting first your right hand and, as soon as there is enough room, your left hand, in front of you. Keep your elbows and hands relaxed throughout.

6 Keeping your hands in the same plane, draw them toward each other slightly as you slowly and gracefully move your arms up until they reach position 2 and the movement has begun again.

Do the movement 3 or 9 continuous times. With each repetition, relax more deeply, allowing the sensations awakened by the movement to spread throughout your body. Breathe very softly through both nose and mouth, belly and chest relaxed. Then adapt the downward movement to bring your hands to rest on your knees.

CLEAR LIGHT

This exercise can relieve ulcers and stomach pain, as well as psychological tensions. Practise it very gently if you are pregnant, have had any sort of back or neck injury, or have had an operation within the past three or four months. At the end of the exercise, sit quietly for five to ten minutes.

1 Sit on the edge of a straight chair with your feet flat on the floor about 6 inches (15cm) apart, the heels pointing toward each other and the toes pointing out. Place your hands either behind you on the chair, fingers pointing backwards, or next to your hips on the side of the chair, fingers pointing forward.

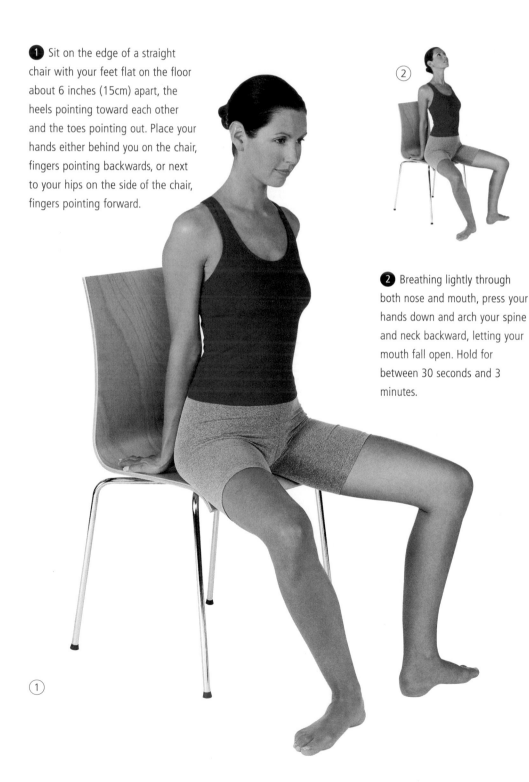

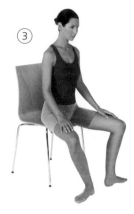

2 Breathing lightly through both nose and mouth, press your hands down and arch your spine and neck backward, letting your mouth fall open. Hold for between 30 seconds and 3 minutes.

3 Slowly straighten your neck and back, sensing the feelings stimulated by the arch. You may feel heat in the back of your neck and at the base of your spine. Sit with your hands on your knees for a few minutes, distributing these sensations throughout your body.

Perform the exercise 3 times.

TOUCHING BODY, MIND AND ENERGY

This exercise increases circulation and awareness, and will invigorate you when you feel tired, sleepy or clumsy. When you finish sit for five minutes or more, sensing the energy flow through your body.

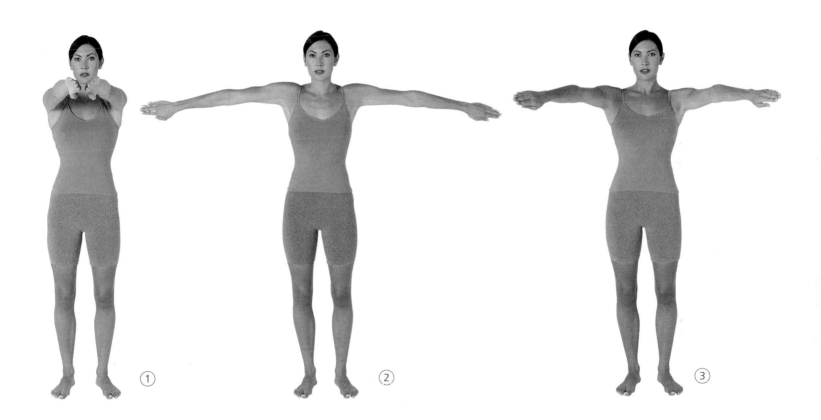

① Stand well-balanced with your feet a comfortable distance apart, your back straight, and your arms relaxed at your sides. Slowly raise your arms in front of you to a little above shoulder-height, with your hands about 2 inches (5cm) apart, the backs of the hands facing each other and the fingers straight.

② Visualize steel bars next to your palms and begin to move your arms slowly out to the sides, as if you were pushing these steel bars apart. Push with strength until your outstretched arms are a little behind your shoulders. Breathe lightly and evenly through both nose and mouth. Keep your belly, chest and thighs relaxed and concentrate lightly on the base of your spine.

③ Imagine the steel bars are by the backs of your hands, and slowly move your hands forward as if you were pushing the bars together. Notice the different quality of the movement in this direction. Feel the energy surrounding your arms while still concentrating loosely on the base of your spine.

Release the tension in your arms slowly, and lower them to your sides. Stand for 2 minutes, expanding the sensations of energy. Perform the entire exercise 3 or 9 times.

If you feel tenseness in the muscles of your upper and middle back, move more gently.

ENERGIZING THE LOWER BODY

This exercise releases energy blockages in the lower body. As you become more familiar with this exercise, try holding the position for longer periods of time. Also try inhaling as you move down and exhaling as you come up. At the end of the exercise, sit in the sitting posture for five to ten minutes, continuing to amplify and extend the sensations in your body.

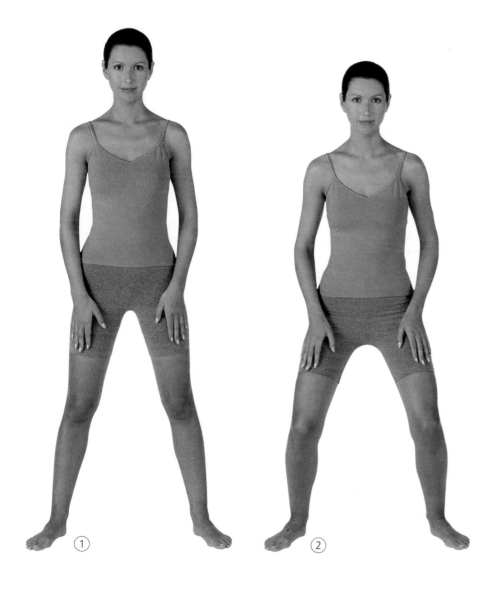

❶ Stand well-balanced with your back straight, your legs wide apart and your toes turned out slightly. Place your hands on your thighs with your thumbs pointing toward the inside of the leg. Breathe softly through both nose and mouth, relax your shoulders, straighten your back and look straight ahead.

❷ Bend your knees and lower your pelvis to the place where energy is strongly activated in your legs (your knees should be bent enough to produce tension in your thighs, but not so much that you feel close to falling backward). If necessary, move up and down a little or move your legs closer or wider apart to find the position. Keep your back straight and your weight evenly distributed. Hold for 15 seconds with your genital and anal areas open and your breathing relaxed and soft.

After 15 seconds slowly straighten your legs, move your feet closer together, relax your arms at your sides and stand or sit for a few minutes, expanding the feelings quickened by the exercise. Perform the exercise 3 times, resting after each repetition.

As you move down during the exercise, you may find that tension prevents you from moving further. Locate the tension, gently release it and continue to lower. Use the exercise to explore subtle tensions that interfere with balance and the even flow of energy in your body.

INNER GOLD

This exercise relieves tension in the stomach area and brings physical openness to the heart area. As you experience this openness you may feel a deep, open, loving feeling that can be distributed to all parts of your body and expanded beyond your body to the surrounding universe. At the end sit in the sitting posture for ten minutes, expanding the sensations stimulated by the exercise.

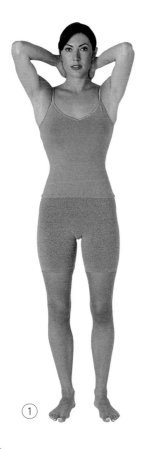

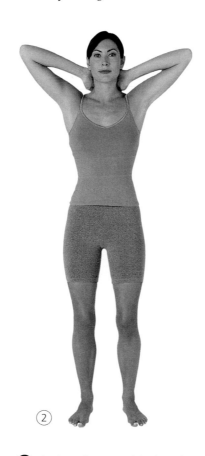

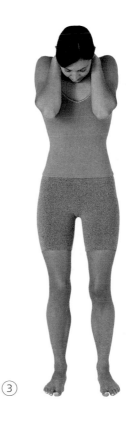

1 Stand well-balanced with your feet about 6 inches (15cm) apart and your back straight. Interlace your fingers and place them at the back of your neck so they support your head.

Perform the movement as slowly as can be coordinated with your breathing.

2 Slowly push your neck back against your hands, spread your elbows apart as wide as possible, bend your knees slightly and lift your chest toward the ceiling. Relax the lower part of your spine while your upper spine arches backward. In this position exhale very slowly and deeply for as long as you can. Feel the stretch in the muscles under your arms and at the sides of your chest. Go deeply into the sensations that arise in your chest.

3 Inhaling, slowly press your hands against the back of your neck; bend your head forward until your chin is near your chest and your elbows hang close together. As you reach this position, hold your breath slightly and relax your shoulders and upper back.

Continuing to inhale, push your neck against your hands, open your elbows and lift your chest toward the ceiling. Exhale in this open position. Perform the movement 3 or 9 times.

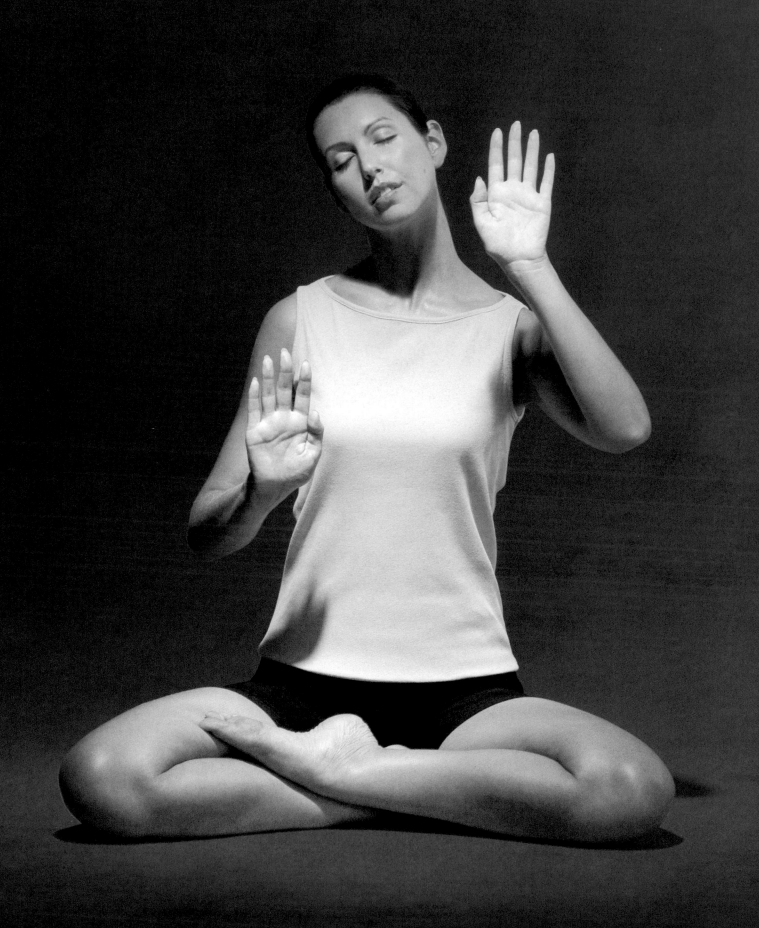

CHAPTER FIVE

BALANCE AND INTEGRATION

*"Balance is a natural condition of flowing feeling
and energy that pervades the entire body and mind."*

We commonly think of balance as our bodily equilibrium or stability. However, this understanding of balance is limited and can be expanded by certain exercises and movements, which show us how to bring our breath, senses and awareness into balance with our bodies and minds. We can make our whole system balanced, for balance is a natural condition of flowing feeling and energy that pervades the entire body and mind. This balance is the objective of Kum Nye. The foundation of balance and the integration of body and mind is relaxation. This chapter helps us to achieve relaxation with a selection of sitting and standing exercises that open us up to new sensory fields and dimensions, expanding our sensations and feelings and thereby bringing body and mind together.

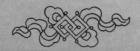

BODY, MIND AND SENSES

*"The foundation of balance and the integration
of body and mind is relaxation."*

People think of relaxation in a variety of ways: as a state of dreaminess; as a strategy for escaping life; as a means to fill in or mark out time. However, true relaxation is the state of perfect balance. When we relax, we open to new sensory fields and dimensions, expanding the sensations and feelings that integrate the body and mind. In this way we learn how to generate and accumulate energy, and use it so that the body and mind work together in a flowing, open way: thoughts and sensations flow smoothly because the mind is clear and vibrant, the body is vital and energetic. During true relaxation there is no longer a self that experiences – we become the experience, totally at one with our bodies, minds and senses.

Faced with the increasing stresses of modern life, many of us find it difficult to find time to relax and open, to bring our awareness to our feelings and the world around us. The result is energy blocks that prevent our minds and bodies from communicating effectively with each other. We become unable to sustain our vitality, concentration or awareness and we function ineffectively, becoming prone to mental and physical imbalances, which are implicated in many illnesses.

The integration and balancing of physical and mental energies that occurs when we practise Kum Nye frees us from these patterns. We learn to flow with experience, allowing it to nourish and satisfy us. Our perspective changes: we become less subject to emotional extremes, understanding that neither good nor bad experiences last for long; we do not try to control or fix our experience because we have learnt to view change positively, seeing it as an opportunity for growth. We develop inner peacefulness, which points us to the harmony of existence so that everything becomes relevant to our lives. We open ourselves to the vital and wholesome nature of all experience, seeing the preciousness and grace of every aspect of life, whether negative or positive.

When our relationship to the world becomes more flowing and complete, our ability to communicate improves and we are less dependent on others to protect our sense of well-being and happiness. As we expand our senses, feelings, thoughts and awareness, we become willing to expand beyond the limitations of our boundaries. Ultimately we learn to tap into the infinite wisdom of the cosmos, which enables us to understand the true beauty, richness and value of our inner resources.

The exercises

The exercises in this chapter are divided into three levels. In terms of difficulty, the exercises in level one and two correspond to the level one and two gentle movement exercises. When approaching the exercises in this chapter for the first time, incorporate them gradually into your existing practice by practising one or two of the balance and integration exercises, alongside a couple of the gentle movement exercises with which you are already familiar. Once you are acquainted with all the exercises you can mix and match them as you choose.

In both this chapter and chapter six there is a progression within each level and from level to level. If you wish try out the exercises in the order that they are presented but do not feel that you must do them in this progression. Certain exercises will suit you better than others so it is fine to do the exercises within a stage in a different sequence or to practise some of the exercises in level two, or even level three, before you have attempted all of the exercises in level one. Feel free to experiment with different combinations of exercises: let your body lead you to those exercises that stimulate the most vital feeling for you and vary the sequence and combination of exercises to ensure that your practice is interesting and balanced.

Continue to allow forty-five minutes a day for your practice. If you cannot spare that much time, twenty to thirty minutes will also bring results. As before, practise two or three movement exercises each day, doing each exercise three or nine times. Choose three or four exercises that you like and work with them until you feel confident that you have touched your feelings deeply. This may take two or three weeks. Then over the next six to eight weeks, work with some of the other level one exercises so that gradually you increase your vocabulary of exercises to approximately ten. Practise some of the standing exercises as well as the sitting ones. Sometimes you may find it helpful to do a sitting or breathing exercise, or perhaps a self-massage, together with the movement exercises.

Some of the exercises in level two and three involve holding a position for a period of time. You can measure the time by counting your outbreaths. Before beginning the exercise, time your breathing for a few minutes so that you can calculate your average number of outbreaths per minute.

While you are in the posture, explore the quality of your holding: let it be as relaxed as possible, without any special purpose. When you release tension after holding, do so very slowly so that you feel more and the sensations quickened by the exercise last as long as possible. The longer a feeling-tone is expanded, the more it can spread beyond the body, stimulating interactions with surrounding space.

As the feelings expand, bring breath, motion, feeling and mind into unity. Balance the breath, balance the senses, balance your awareness, balance your body. Then you will develop a quality in your practice that is free from holding or clinging and you will discover the joy of exercising without effort.

Level one

Most of the exercises in level one release tension in the upper body – the shoulders, chest, back, arms, neck and head. As tensions in these areas lessen, it is possible to feel more in the heart. These exercises also develop valuable healing energies, so it is important to explore some of them quite deeply. They are particularly effective when practised in conjuction with some of the self-massages and gentle movement exercises.

Level two

Many of the level two exercises also release tension in the upper body, balancing inner energies so that feelings flow more freely and the body and mind can make contact with one another. Fully explore each exercise that you select until you are familiar with the range of feelings that it stimulates and its special qualities of balance. Remember not to go too fast or do too much. If you begin to feel overwhelmed by the possibilities opening up to you in these exercises, stay with that feeling and bring it into your practice. Let your self-imposed limitations open into deeper feeling and sensation; allow your energies to expand until you see that all limitations are arbitrary and self-imposed and that your experience can be as large as the universe itself.

Level three

The exercises in this group are a little more difficult than those at lower levels. This does not necessarily mean that the movements of the exercises are physically more demanding (although this is true in some cases). Rather, it means that greater concentration is required to touch and develop the feeling-tones stimulated by the exercises.

After several months of practising Kum Nye, you will probably find that you are ready for the earlier of the level three balance and integration exercises. However, if you get little result from an exercise, you should put it aside and return to it at a later date. Only practise the exercises toward the end of this stage when you have a thorough experience of Kum Nye.

Extending your practice

When you are very familiar with an exercise, try doing it for longer periods of time, up to an hour. Experiment with different tempos and degrees of tension, noticing the different qualities of feeling at various speeds. The exercises that are done tensely can also be done loosely, and similarly those done loosely can also be done tensely. You could also try practising at different times and in different places.

LOOSENING UP THE MIND

*This exercise helps to integrate the mind and body, and is ideal for banishing sluggishness in the morning.
If you are pregnant or have had any kind of neck injury, it is best not to do this exercise. At the end sit
quietly for five to ten minutes, amplifying and extending your sensations and feelings.*

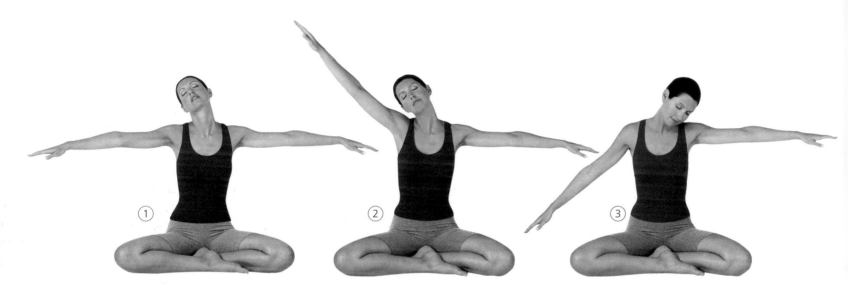

1 Sit cross-legged on a mat or cushion, back straight. Slowly lift your arms away from your sides until they are stretched out at shoulder-height, palms down. Close your eyes. Breathing softly through nose and mouth, slowly rotate your head in a clockwise direction.

This exercise may seem awkward or difficult at first. Your mind may be set in a familiar pattern of movement that you feel unwilling to change. Use the movement to "exercise" feelings of unwillingness until they become a natural flow of feeling and energy. Relax your stomach and let your breath become even. Bring this breath into the movement so the rotations become smooth and spacious.

2 As you complete the first rotation, begin to rotate your right arm up, back, down and forward. Coordinate the 2 circles, making them slow, large and full. Go deeply into the sensations produced. You may feel a delicious warmth in your arms and at the back of your neck. Let the warmth flow down your spine and spread throughout your body.

Make 3 coordinated rotations of the head and right arm; then change the direction of the circles and make 3 more rotations in the other direction. To finish, lower your hands to your knees and rest for a few minutes, continuing to expand your feelings. Repeat the sequence of rotations with the head and the left arm, resting for a few minutes afterward.

3 To complete the exercise, do the whole series of rotations again, but this time with the head and arm moving in opposite directions from each other: when the head moves clockwise, the arm will move forward, down, back and up. Begin with your head and right arm, then rest for a few minutes, hands on knees, before repeating the movement with the head and left arm. Keep your breathing soft and even throughout, uniting it with your sensations.

AWAKENING THE SENSES

This exercise releases tension in the back of the neck, the shoulders, the upper back, and sometimes the lower back. If you are pregnant or have had any kind of neck injury, it is best not to do this exercise. At the end sit in the sitting posture for five to ten minutes, enlarging and deepening the sensations within and around your body.

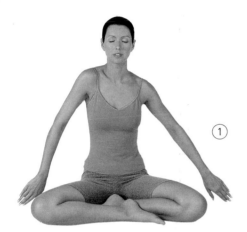 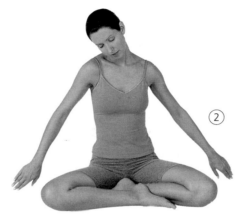 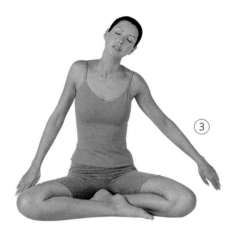

1 Sit cross-legged on a mat or cushion, back straight. Lift your arms away from your sides approximately 6 inches (15cm), palms facing behind you. Ensure your pelvis is high enough to allow your arms to move without your hands touching the floor. Gently close your eyes, and slowly rotate your right shoulder up, back, down and forward.

2 As you complete the first rotation, begin to rotate your head in a clockwise direction. Coordinate the movements, making the circles as full as possible. As you move breathe gently through both nose and mouth, and concentrate lightly on the back of your neck.

Make 3 coordinated rotations, then change the direction of the rotations and continue 3 more times. Then rest briefly, hands on knees, allowing the feelings awakened to flow down your spine and throughout your body. Now repeat the rotations with your left shoulder. After completing these movements, bring your hands to your knees and rest for a few minutes, continuing to expand your sensations.

3 To complete the exercise, do the whole series of rotations again, this time moving the shoulder and head in opposite directions: when the shoulder moves up, back, down and forward, the head moves counterclockwise. Begin with the right shoulder and head, rest for a few minutes, hands on knees, and repeat with the left shoulder and head.

Develop the shape of the movements, paying particular attention to the points when the head and shoulder are in their highest and lowest positions, and nearest to and farthest from each other. Keep in mind the contours of the movement and allow the feelings generated to permeate this shape.

BALANCING THE SENSES

This exercise involves the coordination of three different movements to balance the body, mind and senses.
If you are pregnant or have had any kind of neck injury, it is best not to do this exercise. At the end of the exercise,
sit quietly for five minutes, continuing to expand the sensations within and around your body.

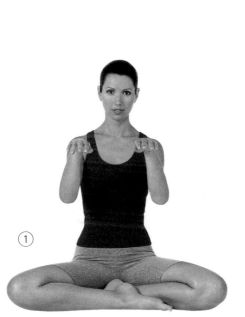 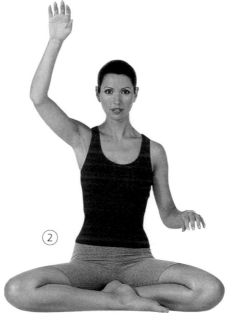 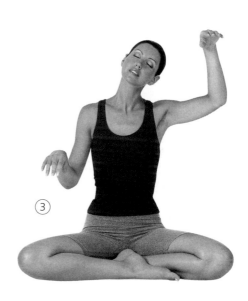

❶ Sit cross-legged on a mat or cushion with your back straight and your hands on your knees. Lift your arms in front of you to chest-height with your elbows loosely bent and your hands relaxed, palms down and fingers pointing forward.

❷ Visualize two large clock faces side by side facing you. Position your left hand at 3 on the left clockface, and your right hand at 9 on the right clockface. Your hands will be approximately 4 inches (10cm) apart. Very slowly draw two large clockwise circles with your hands and arms simultaneously, beginning at 3 and moving toward 6 with the left hand, beginning at 9 and moving toward 12 with the right hand. Make the circles as large as possible without overlapping them.

❸ When you achieve a smooth rhythm, close your eyes and coordinate these movements with a very slow clockwise rotation of your head. Keep your belly relaxed and breathe softly and smoothly through both nose and mouth.

Continue for 2 minutes, then gradually diminish the movement until you are no longer moving. Lower your hands to your knees and sit for 2 minutes, expanding the sensations generated by the movements. Repeat the exercise, making counterclockwise circles with both the arms and the head.

SWIMMING IN SPACE

The first part of this exercise (steps one to three) releases tension in the back, throat, neck and back of the head. The second part (steps four and five) distributes the feelings released in the first part of the exercise throughout the whole body. To complete the exercise, lower your arms to your sides from the overhead position and sit in the sitting posture for five to ten minutes, expanding the sensations quickened by this movement.

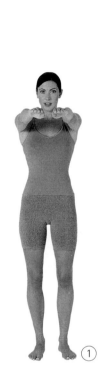 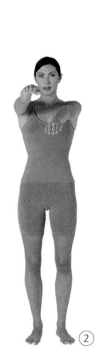 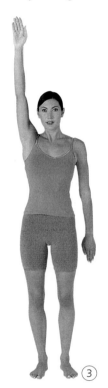 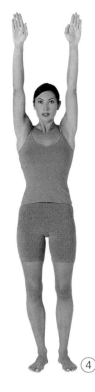 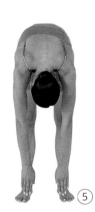

① ② ③ ④ ⑤

❶ Stand well-balanced, feet comfortably spaced, back straight and arms stretched out in front at shoulder-height with the palms down.

❷ Breathing easily through both nose and mouth with your belly relaxed, simultaneously move your right arm up a little and your left arm down a little. Then reverse the movement, raising your left arm and lowering your right arm. Keep your arms and hands straight and relaxed throughout. Move very slowly.

❸ Gradually extend the movement until each arm moves up and down as far as it can go. Pay attention to the particular sense of space awakened by this exercise; you may feel a quality akin to that of swimming. Continue the full movement of the arms for 3 to 5 minutes.

Slowly decrease the range of the movement until your arms are still and extended in front of you at shoulder-height. Slowly lower them to your sides and stand quietly for a few minutes, expanding your sensations and feelings.

❹ Slowly lift your arms in front of you until they are overhead with the palms facing forward. Keep your arms parallel to each other and straight.

❺ Moving your arms, head and torso together, bend down from the waist until your fingers almost touch the floor.

Then swing up slowly until your back is straight and your arms are outstretched overhead. Continue this slow swinging movement, down and up, 3 or 9 times. Keep your arms straight throughout.

INTEGRATING BODY AND MIND

This exercise releases tension in the neck, head, shoulders, chest and spine, and balances their interconnecting energies. It is best not to do this exercise if you are pregnant. Perform it gently if you have had a neck or back injury or an operation within three or four months. Rest for five to ten minutes at the end of the exercise.

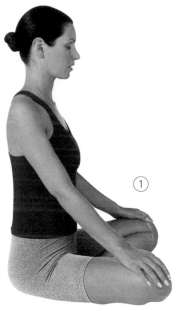
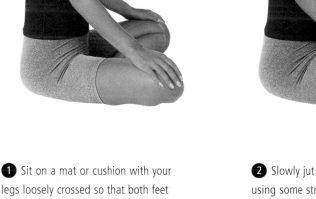
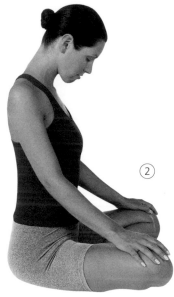
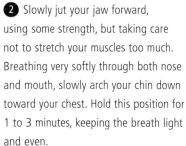
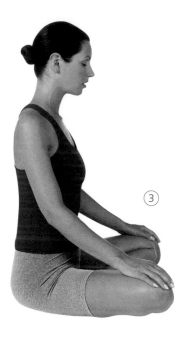

❶ Sit on a mat or cushion with your legs loosely crossed so that both feet rest on the mat or the floor. Place your hands on your knees, lift your shoulders a little and move them back slightly so your arms straighten.

❷ Slowly jut your jaw forward, using some strength, but taking care not to stretch your muscles too much. Breathing very softly through both nose and mouth, slowly arch your chin down toward your chest. Hold this position for 1 to 3 minutes, keeping the breath light and even.

❸ Slowly lift your chin and very slowly release the tension in your jaw, neck and shoulders, sensing the subtle qualities of feeling that arise. Let these feelings be distributed throughout your body.

Rest for a few minutes, then repeat the exercise 2 more times, resting for several minutes after each repetition.

Each time you finish the exercise, gently loosen the neck muscles. Slowly move your head forward and back, from side to side (looking left to right), so your ear moves toward your shoulder. Then massage your neck gently.

INTERACTING BODY AND MIND

This exercise relieves headaches and tension in the back, shoulders and legs. When you finish sit in the sitting posture for five to ten minutes, expanding the sensations stimulated by the movement.

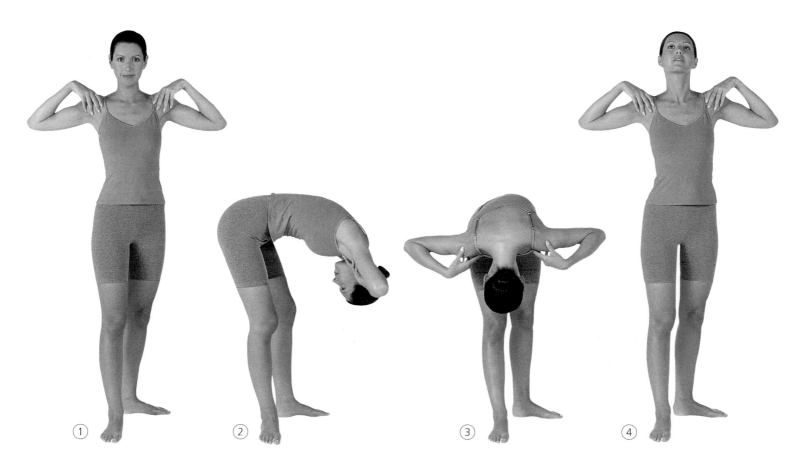

1 Stand well-balanced, legs comfortably spaced, back straight and arms relaxed at your sides. Turn your left foot out so the toes point to the left and place your right foot about 12 inches (30cm) in front of you, toes pointing forward and the heel on a line with the heel of the left foot. Lift your arms to shoulder-height and place your hands on your shoulders, fingers on the front of the shoulders and thumbs on the back. Press down with as much contact between hand and shoulder as possible.

2 In this position, eyes open, very slowly begin to rotate your upper torso. Leading with your left elbow, turn your torso to the left as far as you can go without straining, then bend down to the side, letting your head hang.

3 Without stopping or raising your torso, continue the rotation to the right.

4 When you have rotated as far as you can to the right, slowly straighten up on your right side. As you come up, look upward.

Perform 3 or 9 of these slow rotations, breathing easily through both nose and mouth, and pressing your hands against your shoulders throughout. Then reverse the position of your feet and do 3 or 9 rotations on the other side, leading the turning of the torso with your right elbow.

VITALIZING ENERGY

This exercise boosts energy levels on a mental as well as physical level.
Practise this exercise when you are feeling tired or run-down. At the end sit in the sitting posture
for five to ten minutes, expanding the feelings quickened by the exercise.

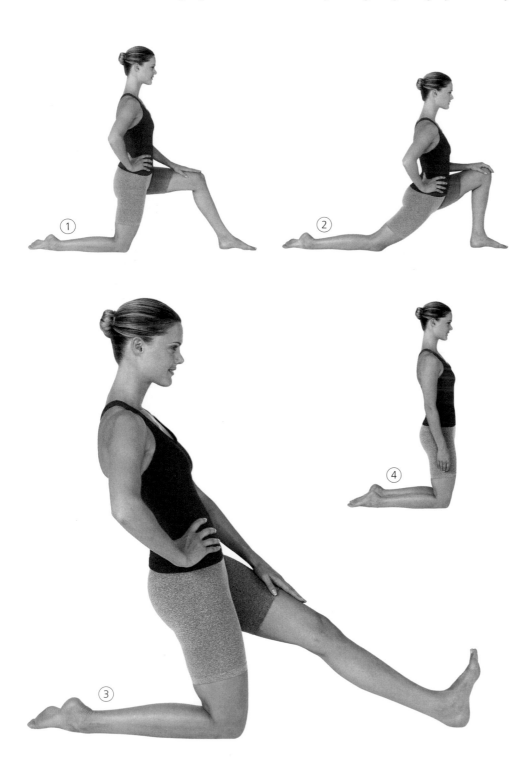

1 Kneel on your right knee with the toes pointing behind you. Bend the left knee and place your left foot on the floor as far in front of you as possible. Place your right hand on your right hip, and your left hand on your left knee.

2 Face forward with your back straight. Keeping your left foot in the same place, shift your weight forward and increase the bend in your left knee until you feel a stretch in both thighs. Make sure your legs are wide apart. Relax your arms, hands and chest, and hold this position for about 30 seconds, breathing gently through both nose and mouth and feeling the sensations produced by the stretch.

3 Very slowly shift your weight back onto your right leg, straighten your left leg and flex your left ankle so that your toes point to the ceiling. Attend to the subtle qualities of feeling that arise as you perform this leg stretch.

4 Slowly relax your left leg and foot, and kneel on both knees. Rest briefly, continuing to feel the sensations stimulated by the stretches.

Now reverse the position of the legs and hands and perform the exercise on the other side. Do the complete exercise, first on one side, then on the other, 3 times, resting briefly after each repetition.

LOOSENING UP THE SELF-IMAGE

This exercise stimulates the skin and activates new mental and muscular patterns.
At the end of the exercise, sit in the sitting posture for five to ten minutes,
expanding the sensations stimulated by the movement.

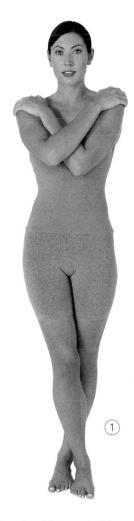

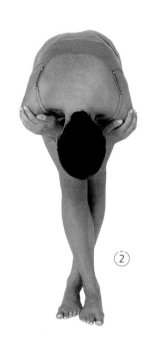

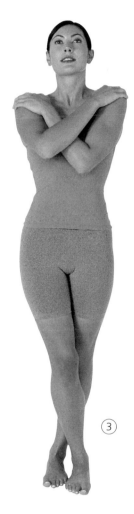

To extend this exercise, try it 3 times with the legs crossed left over right and the arms crossed right over left. Reverse the position of both arms and legs and repeat 3 more times. Then sit for 5 to 10 minutes.

①

②

③

❶ Stand well-balanced with your back straight and your arms relaxed at your sides. Cross your arms in front of your chest, the right over the left, and hold your shoulders with your hands, letting the elbows hang down. Cross the right leg over the left and place your right foot next to the left foot.

❷ In this position, breathing gently through both nose and mouth, very slowly bend forward from the waist as low as possible without straining, allowing your head to hang.

❸ Very slowly rise up and arch backward slightly, focusing on your feet.

Do the movement 3 or 9 times in this position. Then cross the left arm over the right, and the left leg over the right, and repeat the exercise 3 or 9 times. Notice the different qualities of feeling stimulated by the change in position.

BALANCING MIND AND SENSES

This exercise stimulates several different kinds of energy in the lower body and improves balance.
It also develops an awareness of the body and its relationship to its surroundings.
At the end sit for five to ten minutes, expanding the feelings quickened by the exercise.

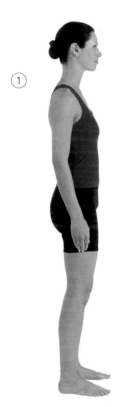

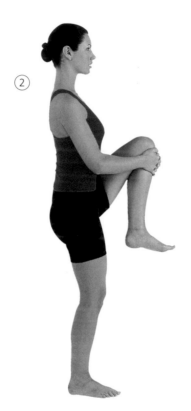

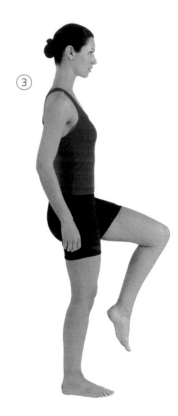

❶ Stand with your feet slightly apart, your back straight, your arms at your sides and your body balanced.

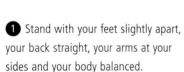

Throughout the exercise let your attitude be casual and unambitious so that you can be sensitive to subtle muscular and energetic changes – by sensing the moments at which certain muscles take over a movement, we learn to combine relaxation and controlled movement.

❷ Slowly bend your left knee, clasp it with interlaced hands, draw it up toward your chest and flex your left ankle. Relax your pelvis and move your shoulders back a little. Look straight ahead with soft eyes, and balance casually in this position for 1 to 3 minutes, breathing gently through both nose and mouth. At first hold your leg tightly with your hands, then slowly release the holding (without moving the leg) until your hands become relaxed, keeping your chest relaxed as you do so.

❸ Keeping your hands around your knee, slowly lower your left leg to the point at which control of the movement can pass easily to your leg. Then open your hands and slowly lower your leg, noticing the feeling-tones that arise just before your foot touches the ground.

Do the complete movement, first on one side, then the other, 3 or 9 times.

COORDINATING BODY AND MIND

This exercise improves the circulation of blood on a physical level and energy on an energetic level. It also develops the focus of the mind and the coordination of the body. At the end of the exercise, roll onto your back and rest for five to ten minutes. Use the resting time to go deeper into the sensations activated by the movement.

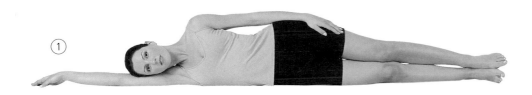

1 Lie on your right side, your left leg on top of the right, with your right arm extended along the floor above your head, palm down. Rest your head on your right arm and place your left arm along the side of your body, palm down. Make sure your body is lying in a straight line.

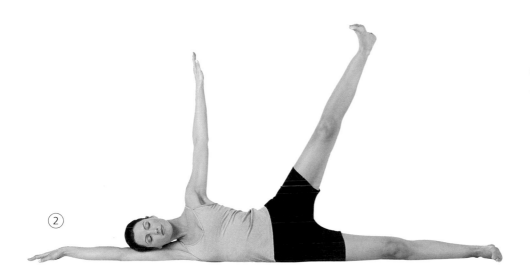

2 Keeping your legs straight, flex both ankles so your toes point toward your head. Slowly stretch both your left arm and leg as if to lengthen them. Then, continuing the stretch and keeping the ankles flexed, slowly lift your left arm and leg until the arm is vertical and the leg is as high as it will comfortably go. Coordinate this movement so that both the arm and the leg cover the distance in the same amount of time, breathing gently and evenly through both nose and mouth throughout.

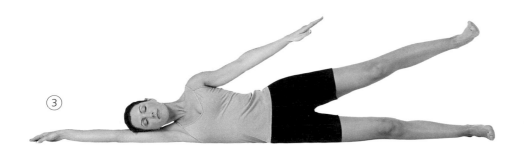

3 Moving as slowly as you can so that you feel more, gently lower both your arm and leg, while continuing the stretch.

Perform the exercise 3 times on each side, resting after each repetition.

COORDINATING THE WHOLENESS OF ENERGY

This exercise increases coordination. It develops the muscles of the legs and stimulates the flow of energy from the legs, through the back, to the head. At the end of the exercise, sit in the sitting posture for five to ten minutes, expanding the feelings generated by the movement.

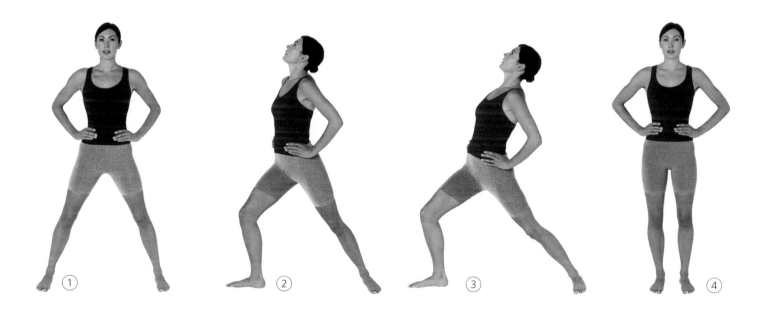

❶ Stand with your back straight, your feet wide apart and pointed straight ahead, and your hands on your hips. Your body and mind should be balanced and focused.

❷ Turn your right foot to the right until it is at a right angle to your left foot, bend your right knee, and turn your torso to the right so you face the same direction as your right foot. Keep your back and left leg straight. With your head back, chin in, chest high and elbows out, look at a spot on the wall in front of you, near the ceiling. Relax your belly and breathe smoothly through both nose and mouth.

❸ Keeping your back and left leg straight, lower your body by increasing the bend in your right knee and relaxing your pelvis. Lower until you reach a place of tension and energy. See how you feel at different points as you go down, and let your feelings guide you to the place where sensation is strongest. When you find this place, hold until you begin to shake.

If you find position 3 difficult to hold at first, move down and up slowly several times until you become more familiar with the sensation of tension in the right knee and leg. Then try holding the position for a few seconds.

❹ Slowly return to an upright position. Turn your right toes and torso to the left so that you again face forward and move your feet closer together. Breathe softly and evenly so that the different steps flow smoothly into each other.

Repeat the exercise on the left side. Do the entire exercise, on both sides, 3 times.

Throughout the exercise keep the movements flowing smoothly and stay in touch with your feelings. Do not let the movements become mechanical.

TRANSFORMING EMOTIONS

This exercise improves circulation and stimulates the release of hormones and the flow of energies in the lower body. Although our emotions tend to throw us off-balance, in this exercise, we use the energy of strong emotions, such as resentment, to keep us balanced, rather than dissipating the energy through negativity. If the position is held for long enough, pure energy flows throughout the body.

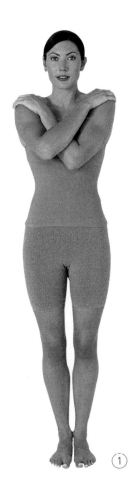

①

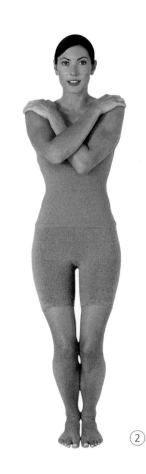

②

❶ Cross your arms in front of your chest and hold your shoulders with your hands, keeping your elbows down.

❷ Legs together, heels on the floor, back straight, slowly bend at the knees. Maintain internal balance as you lower, without tensing up. Well above a full squat you will discover a place of balance and energy. Move up and down a little to find the right place. You may feel heat rise in your body and begin to shake. Remain with these sensations and hold for 1 to 5 minutes, concentrating on the energy in your spine.

Slowly return to a standing position, releasing the tension. Stand with your arms at your sides for 3 to 5 minutes; then repeat the exercise twice, standing or sitting after each repetition. Then sit in the sitting posture for 10 to 15 minutes, expanding the sensations generated by the movement.

As you do the exercise, search out the inner tensions that throw you off-balance and release them. Feel for any memory that makes you tense and relax the sensations associated with that memory. Breathe softly and gently into places of blockage. If an emotion is so strong that the tightness manifests as pain, breathe into the pain until the holding relaxes and you discover a kernel of new energy. Keep your stomach relaxed so that energy rising up from the legs can flow through your spine and be distributed to your whole body. With practice the exercise may become effortless.

When you have gone down a certain distance in this position, you may find that tightness prevents you from going further, and you are beginning to lift your heels from the floor. Stop and locate the tension – it may be in your pelvis or legs. Let it go and continue to lower, keeping your back straight.

OPENING THE HEART

*This exercise opens the heart centre, improves breathing and circulation,
and massages internal muscles. At the end of the exercise, sit quietly in the sitting posture
for five to ten minutes and taste the quality of the relaxation that arises.*

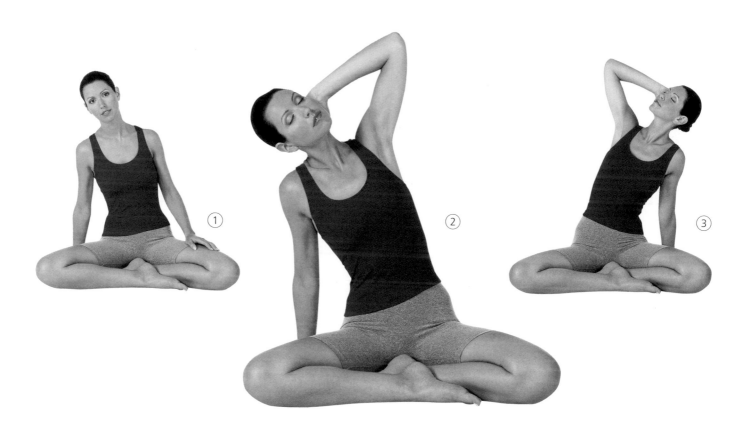

❶ Sit cross-legged on a mat or cushion and support yourself with your right hand placed on the floor, a comfortable distance away from you. Ensure that your hand is not too far in front of you or behind you.

❷ Place your left hand over your left ear, elbow up. In this position, slowly arch to the right, keeping your right arm straight. Support yourself firmly with your right hand so that you can maximize and balance the arching of your left side. Keep your knees down as much as possible. Allow your ribs to lift away from your pelvis, opening like a fan; let space expand within the bones of your hip and ribs, and in the muscles under your arm. Hold this position for 1 to 3 minutes, breathing softly and evenly through both nose and mouth.

❸ Release the stretch very slowly – take about 1 minute for this – feeling the sensations generated by holding this position. Then place your right hand over your right ear, support yourself with your left hand on the floor beside you, and arch slowly to the left.

Do the complete exercise, first on one side and then the other, 3 or 9 times.

INCREASING ENDURANCE

This exercise balances the energy of the body, and develops our ability to stay balanced during critical points of emotional or psychological change. At the end sit for five to ten minutes, expanding the feelings stimulated by the exercise.

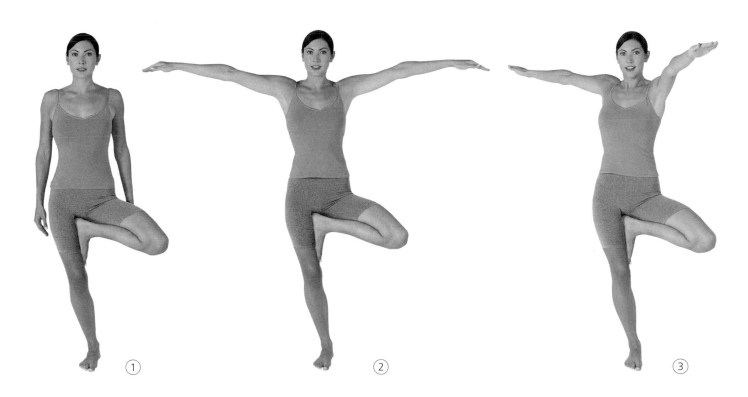

①   ②   ③

1 Balance on your right leg with the sole of your left foot pressed against your upper right thigh, your heel near the crotch, and your left knee out to the side. Lightly press your heel against your thigh to help keep the left foot in place.

2 Without effort, slowly lift your arms away from your sides, letting them float up until they are extended slightly above shoulder-height, with the palms down.

3 Slowly turn at the waist to the right, and then to the left, keeping your head still and looking straight ahead. Breathe lightly and evenly, keeping your body loose and and your stomach relaxed.

Lower your arms and leg simultaneously, sensing the subtle changes in feeling as you come to balance on both feet. Stand for a minute. You may feel a release of tension in the neck and shoulders and a balanced feeling throughout your torso. Reverse the position of the legs, and repeat on the other side. Do the complete movement 3 or 9 times.

EMBRACING SPACE

*This exercise develops awareness of the energies that surround us and our relationship to those energies.
You can perform this exercise either standing on one or both legs, or sitting. When you finish stand silently on
both feet for several minutes, your arms relaxed at your sides; then sit for five to ten minutes. You may
feel a deep calm within your bones, especially the bones of your arms and chest.*

1 Balance on your right leg with the sole of your left foot pressed against your upper right thigh and your left knee out to the side. Slowly lift your arms to shoulder-height in front of you and then cross them, holding the arms tightly just above the elbow.

2 Slowly raise your arms over and a little behind your head, stretching upward. Let your neck settle down between your shoulders. Slowly look toward the ceiling, open your mouth, and stretch a little more. Balance casually in this position. Loosen your stomach muscles; you may then find that you can stretch a little more. Your upper back may be slightly arched.

3 Now slowly unfold your arms, with the palms facing toward the ceiling, until your arms straighten overhead.

4 In a slow, uninterrupted motion, lower your arms to your sides. Allow your hands and chest to open.

When your arms reach your sides, slowly lower your leg to the floor, until you are standing on both feet. Notice the sensations just before your foot touches the floor. Now reverse the position of your legs and repeat the movement. This time inhale slowly as you stretch your tightly crossed arms upward. Hold the inhalation for a few seconds, then exhale as you open your arms upward, continuing to exhale as your arms float down to your sides. Do the complete exercise 3 times, coordinating your breathing with the movement.

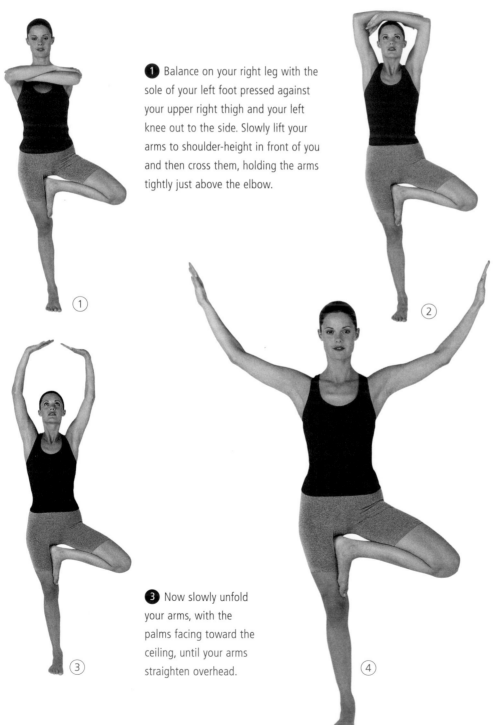

INCREASING INNER BALANCE

This exercise gives inner balance to both the upper and lower body. At the end rest on your back (with your knees bent if you wish) for five minutes, continuing to expand the sensations stimulated by the exercise.

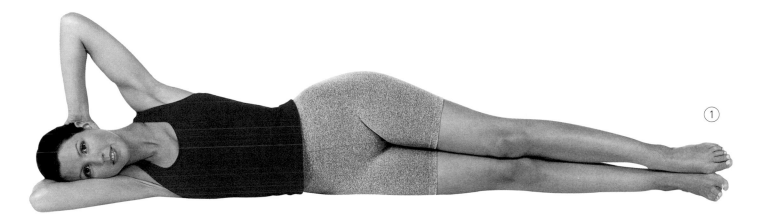

① Lie on your right side with your legs straight, the left leg on top of the right. Interlace your fingers and place them behind your head so that your head rests on your right arm and your left elbow points to the ceiling.

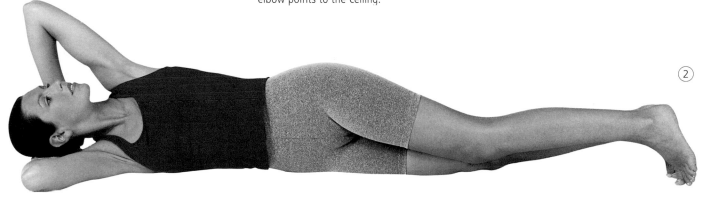

② Slowly begin to stretch, moving your left hip toward the floor in front of you and moving your left elbow to the left until you are looking up at the ceiling and your left shoulder comes near the floor. As your hip moves forward, your legs may turn so that you can place your weight on your toes. Move easily without straining; it does not matter how far you stretch. Hold the stretch for 30 seconds to 1 minute, breathing softly through both your nose and mouth, and gently increasing the stretch as subtle tensions are released.

Slowly return to the original position, expanding the sensations awakened by the stretch. Now roll onto your left side, and repeat the stretch. Notice on which side of your body the stretch is easier. Do the complete exercise, on the right and left, 3 times.

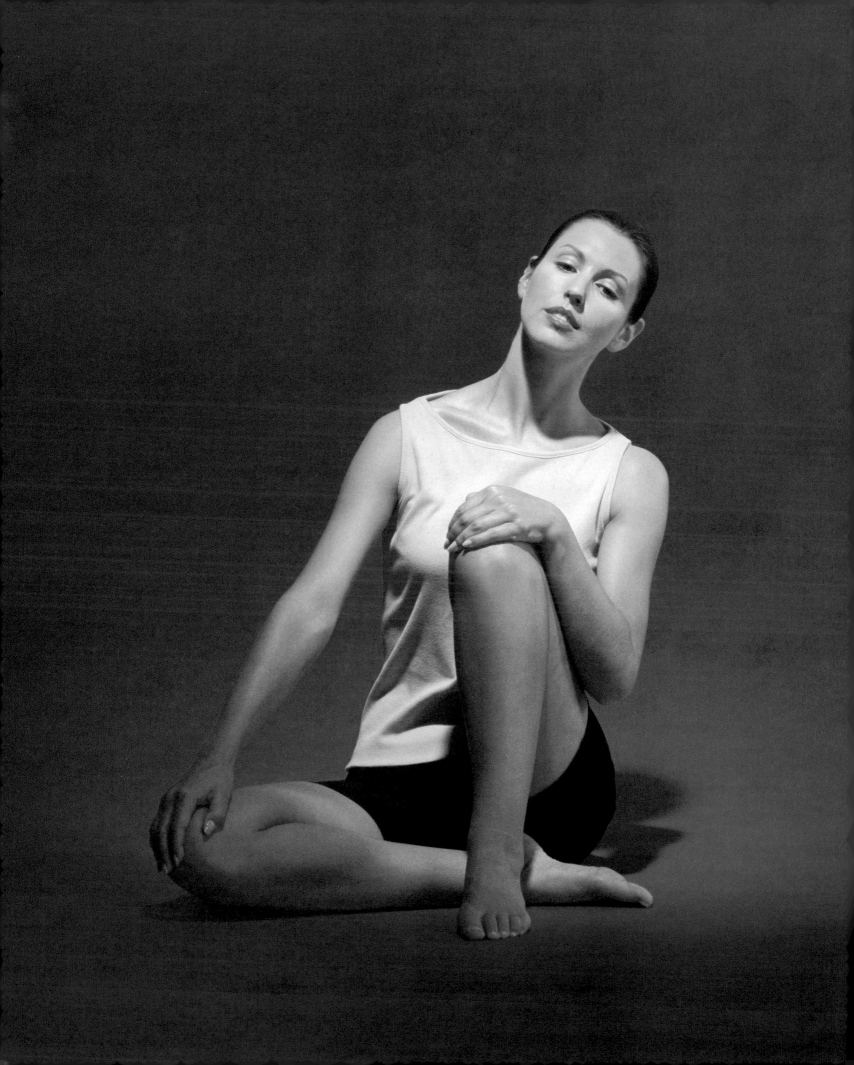

CHAPTER SIX

STIMULATION AND TRANSFORMATION

"As we move and experience, even as we breathe, the energies within and around us continuously interact."

We have contacted the subtle energies of the body and used them to balance and integrate the mind and body. The exercises in this chapter take the process of Kum Nye one stage further, using the subtle energies of the body to stimulate energies at deeper levels of being — transforming blockages and negative energies into free-flowing neutral energy at emotional and ultimately spiritual levels of being. Once we penetrate through to this neutral energy of the cosmos we begin to experience wholeness — a perception of oneness and a sense of connection with our surroundings that is the aim of Kum Nye. The exercises in this chapter are organised according to three levels of difficulty and provide a complement to the exercises of the previous chapter; together these two chapters take us to advanced levels of practice and understanding.

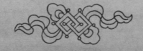

ENERGIES OF LIFE

"The body is like a vessel filled and surrounded by space.
The whole body exercises in space."

Energy is continuously being channelled through our bodies, from cell to cell, between our minds and our bodies, as well as between ourselves and the world around us. As we move and experience, even as we breathe, the energies within and around us continuously interact. We tend to think of energy and matter as being opposites, but even the most solid objects are actually made up of moving energies: matter and energy are equivalent on all levels. Our physical bodies are much less solid than they seem; rather than being fixed and impervious objects, they are essentially flowing and open, participating in an ongoing process of embodiment of energies.

When these energies are flowing smoothly, we have access to an abundance of energy, the body becomes healthy, the mind clear and the senses vital as every aspect of our being regenerates. Feelings of love and openness nourish us and radiate into the surrounding environment. All our experience participates in this ongoing process of enjoyment and embodiment.

When we obstruct this completely open flow, slowing the energies down and misdirecting them, our experience becomes contracted. We freeze our sensations by concentrating on our thoughts about them, instead of experiencing our sensations directly, letting them flow to our hearts where they deepen into nourishing joy and satisfaction. We become like bees, tapping beautiful flowers for pollen, but never enjoying the sweetness of the honey.

Having cut off our inner sources of sensation and satisfaction, we look for them outside ourselves, directing our energies outward. We fill our minds with ideas and expectations of what we want for the future instead of enjoying what is at hand. We skim over the surface of our true feelings, instead directing energy into our emotions in an attempt to feel more. In contrast to the depth and stability of feelings, emotions are superficial and constantly in flux. They quickly and easily feed us strong sensations, but these sensations are imbalanced and cannot truly satisfy us – they stir up dissatisfaction instead of fulfilment. The resulting psychological tensions then manifest themselves on a physical level, automatically producing more tightening, which is reflected in negative patterns of thought, feeling and action.

As our ability to contact our senses diminishes, so too does our vitality. In response we may seek to conserve our energy by relying on energy-saving devices, such as washing machines, which are powered by electricity. However, this reliance on external forms of energy only serves to undermine our health further. We then try to heal ourselves in an orthodox manner, treating our bodies as an object that is separate from ourselves and thereby reinforcing rather than healing the damaging schism between body and mind. What we often fail to realize is that the remedy lies in the integration of our bodies and minds. As we have seen, we can achieve this by stimulating and expanding our sensations and feelings until ultimately we are able to transform all energies, whether negative or positive, into the pure neutral energy of the cosmos.

Contact with this pure neutral energy often occurs during the more advanced stages of Kum Nye practice (although it can take place at any time). When this happens, we begin to work with the subtlest energetic level of the body and it becomes possible to experience the opening of energy centres. When the head centre opens it becomes easy to think and communicate clearly, and visionary powers become possible; when the throat centre opens intuitive powers develop, revealing to us the symbolic world of poetry and art; when the heart centre opens, the perceived separation between ourselves and others dissolves and we become a part of everything; when the navel centre opens, craving and grasping cease and a quality of energy akin to heat warms the whole body.

The exercises

As in the balance and integration exercises in the previous chapter, these exercises are grouped into three levels. Each level is equivalent in terms of difficulty to the corresponding levels in the previous chapters. Feel free to move back and forth between the chapters, exploring the exercises of any given level. Alternatively, you may want to explore some of the level two and three exercises in this chapter before completing all of the exercises on the first level.

Simply allow your body and your feelings to guide you in your selection of exercises and the order in which you practise them. However, if you find that you are racing through the exercises without exploring any of them deeply, slow down and follow the progression of exercises given here. Remember to do each exercise completely – either three or nine times and, when appropriate, on both sides of the body.

Level one

The exercises in this stage are all simple to do. Do them slowly, paying sensitive attention to the sensations that occur throughout your whole body. The exercise entitled "Feeling Embodiment" (see p.118), is particularly important for learning to contact the sublest energetic level of the body, for when practised regularly over a period of at least one week, this exercise greatly increases awareness of the energy centres. As these centres become more open, a warm, gentle, deeply satisfying feeling begins to nurture and sustain you. This is the pure energy of the cosmos. As your contact with this energy deepens, its harmonious effect nurtures those around you as well.

Level two

These exercises activate energies in many specific areas of the body, including the hands, wrists, arms, chest, shoulders, back, thighs, legs and toes. As you perform them, distribute the sensations that are awakened in a particular place throughout your entire body until your whole being participates in the internal energy massage. You will probably find that the exercises that lengthen the muscles along the spine release particularly joyful sensations.

Explore any tight areas in your body and mind, but without dwelling on them. The exercise entitled "Transforming Energy" (see p.123) is ideal for working with such tensions, for releasing them through transformation. With continued practice of Kum Nye, tensions melt away, stimulating energy to flow evenly throughout the body in a constant cycle of refreshment.

Level three

These exercises are generally more advanced than those in levels one and two: some are physically quite strenuous; others demand a certain quality of concentration for developing the feeling-tones that the exercise stimulates. You should therefore wait until you have deepened your experience of Kum Nye over a period of several months before you try these exercises. Then, when you feel ready, add one or two of these exercises to your practice. However, do not push yourself. It may take some time before you are ready to attempt these exercises, particularly the last three which are the most difficult.

Extending your practice

If you have not already done so, you might now want to practise some of the exercises at different tempos. Begin with an exercise that you know well and try it in different ways. First perform the exercise slowly, then, without losing touch with the feeling-tones, build up a little speed. Try to develop the different feeling-tones generated at the different tempos.

As in chapter five, all of the exercises in this chapter that are done tensely can be done in a relaxed way, and vice versa. As your awareness of subtle inner feelings grows, you will gradually discover how to use both tempo and tension to strengthen and expand the feeling-tones of each exercise.

However your practice of Kum Nye develops it should always be an open-ended journey into your inner feelings. As your body and mind become more integrated, your experience of greater balance will itself become your guide.

CLEARING CONFUSION

This exercise energizes the navel centre and clears confusion from the mind.
At the end of the exercise, sit quietly for five to ten minutes.

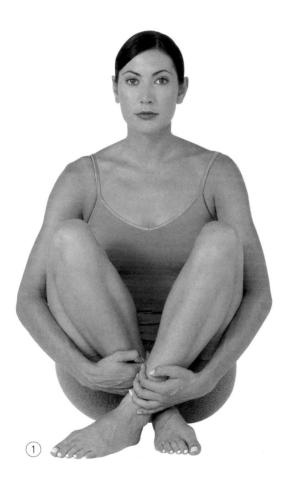

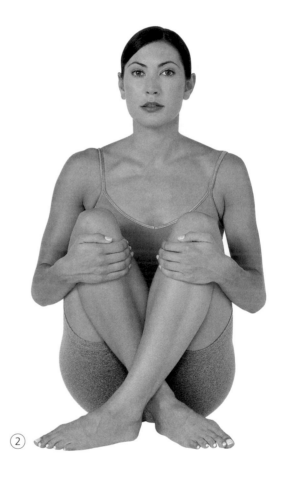

1 Sit on a rug or a flat mat and cross your legs by taking hold of your right ankle with your right hand and your left ankle with your left hand, and drawing your feet along the floor, bringing them as close to your body as you can.

2 Place your hands just below the kneecaps and draw your knees into your chest, keeping your back straight and shoulders down. If possible touch your knees to your chest. Look ahead and hold for 1 to 3 minutes, breathing softly through both nose and mouth, and concentrating lightly on your stomach.

Taking about 1 minute, very slowly release the tension, feeling the sensations that arise. Sit in the sitting posture for a few minutes, exploring these sensations. Repeat the exercise, reversing the position of the legs. Do the entire exercise 3 or 9 times, sitting for a few minutes after each repetition.

RELEASING TENSION

*This exercise releases tension in the neck, shoulders and head; it can relieve headaches.
At the end of the exercise, sit in the sitting posture for five to ten minutes,
continuing to expand the sensations generated by the stretch.*

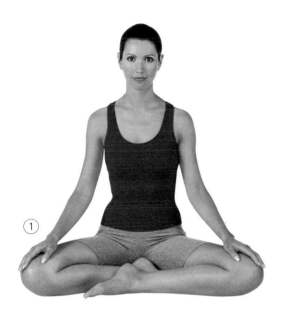

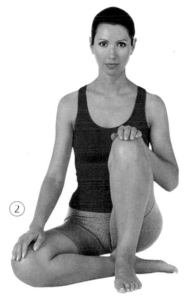

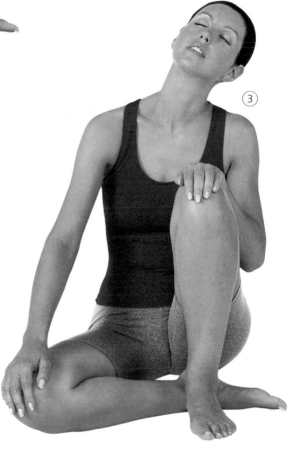

1 Sit on a mat or cushion with your legs loosely crossed, the left leg outside the right.

2 Raise your left knee and bring your left heel in front of your right ankle with the sole of your left foot flat on the floor or mat. Draw your feet as close to your body as you can and place your hands on your knees.

3 Very slowly and gently stretch your neck back and to the left so that your right arm straightens and your head and neck come into a line with your right arm. Keep the right knee down. Hold the diagonal stretch for about 30 seconds, breathing gently and evenly through both nose and mouth.

Take 30 seconds to 1 minute to release the tension. Let your breath and awareness flow with the sensations awakened in your body. Sit quietly for a few minutes. Then reverse the position of your legs and stretch your neck toward the other side. Do the complete exercise 3 or 9 times, resting for a few minutes after each side.

FEELING EMBODIMENT

This exercise develops the kind of concentration that encourages energy to flow, with the result that calm feelings arise and thoughts slow down. Do this exercise on three consecutive days. On the third day alter the quality of the concentration so it becomes less forceful and there is simply a quality of awareness. After concentrating on the navel centre for three days, repeat this exercise with the heart centre, throat centre and head centre (between the eyes), spending three days on each.

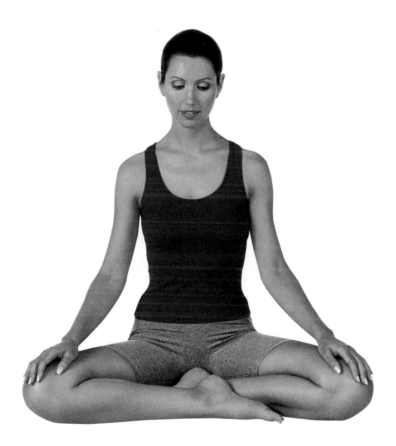

As you practise this exercise you will find that, at times, the feelings that arise are soft and gentle like warm milk — very thick, rich and deep. Become very still and expand these feelings; this will prolong them. Like the breath of a warm summer breeze in a hot place, the feelings heal you within and without, passing through many layers of your body: through your skin, in and between surface tissues and nerves; then deeper to nerves, tissues and organs. Sometimes the feelings move deep within like a little whirl of wind. Feel them as much as you can and distribute them to all the different parts of your body — up to your face and neck, and down to your feet and toes. Subtly hold the breath, just a little tightly, in the lower part of the stomach and in the sacrum; then expand the feelings more and more, until it seems as if the whole universe becomes those feelings.

Sit comfortably in the sitting posture. Concentrate on the energy centre below the navel for half an hour, eyes half-open, or closed if you prefer. Breathe gently and evenly through both nose and mouth.

If you want to practise this exercise over a longer period of time, concentrate on each energy centre for half an hour a day for 2 or 3 weeks before moving on to the next. It should take you between 8 and 12 weeks to go through all four centres. During this time, certain experiences may occur: you may see different objects, or coloured light, such as green, white, red, orange, blue, or perhaps a mixture of colours; you may feel various feeling-tones, or hear high-pitched sounds. If you experience these or other phenomena, do not become attached to or fascinated by them. Just allow them to happen and expand the sensations as much as possible.

If too many thoughts make it difficult for you to sleep, concentrate lightly on the heart centre for half an hour every evening for 2 weeks. Try not to think about anything; just deepen and expand the feeling in your heart centre until a joyful quality develops.

NURTURING SATISFACTION

This exercise increases muscle strength in the arms and relieves tension in the upper body. It can also be done standing. At the end of the exercise, sit quietly in the sitting posture for five to ten minutes, continuing to expand the sensations in your body. You may feel an opening in your chest and upper back, and your breathing may become more open and free-flowing.

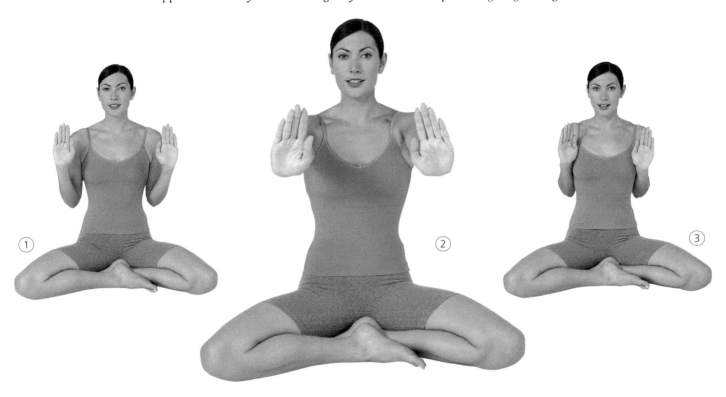

1 Sit cross-legged on a mat or cushion with your hands on your knees. Bend your arms at the elbow, lifting your hands until they are directly in front of your shoulders with the palms facing forward.

2 Imagine that a great force is pushing against your hands. Moving your hands slowly away from your body, push against the force. Allow strong tension to build up in your hands and arms but relax your stomach and lower back, breathing lightly through both nose and mouth. Push against this force until your arms are stretched out in front of you.

3 Without releasing the tension – as if the force is more powerful than you – slowly move your arms back in front of your shoulders, keeping your stomach relaxed. Take about 1 minute to release the tension, noting the sensations in your arms, chest and body, and the qualities of different stages of relaxation.

Then slowly lower your hands to your knees and rest briefly, continuing to expand the feelings stimulated by producing and releasing tension in this way. Do the exercise 3 times, resting briefly after each repetition.

BUILDING STRENGTH
AND CONFIDENCE

*This exercise is ideal for those times when you are feeling weak and vulnerable. In addition to trying
the variations shown opposite, you can also experiment by placing your hands,
once they are heated, on other parts of your body.*

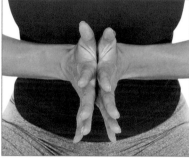

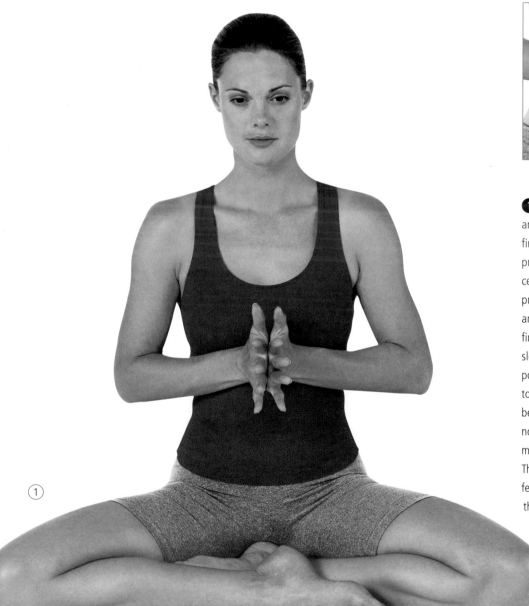

①

1 Sit cross-legged on a mat or cushion and press your palms together with the fingers pointing straight ahead; then press the heels of your hands into the centre of your chest. Keeping your palms pressed tightly together, your elbows out and your shoulders down, separate your fingers and thumbs from each other and slowly move them as far apart as possible. Be sure to press the palms together as you do this and relax your belly. Breathing softly through both nose and mouth, hold this position for 3 minutes, until your palms become heated. Then very slowly release the tension, feeling the sensations that arise. Now do the exercise again, this time holding the position for 5 minutes, separating your fingers and thumbs as much as possible.

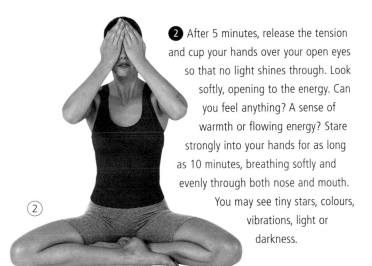

2 After 5 minutes, release the tension and cup your hands over your open eyes so that no light shines through. Look softly, opening to the energy. Can you feel anything? A sense of warmth or flowing energy? Stare strongly into your hands for as long as 10 minutes, breathing softly and evenly through both nose and mouth. You may see tiny stars, colours, vibrations, light or darkness.

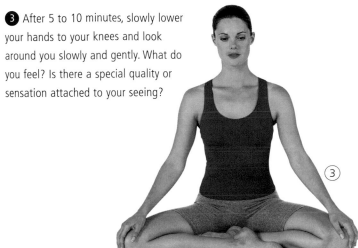

3 After 5 to 10 minutes, slowly lower your hands to your knees and look around you slowly and gently. What do you feel? Is there a special quality or sensation attached to your seeing?

Once your palms are heated, try the following variations:

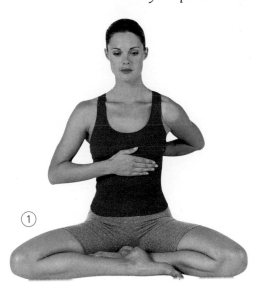

1 Heat up your palms again, holding for 5 minutes, then put one hand cross-wise on your chest and the other cross-wise on the middle of your back. Let the whole hand come in contact with your body. Feel the warmth penetrate your chest and spine as if you had no skin.

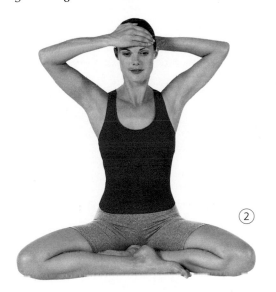

2 After a few minutes, bring one hand to your forehead and the other to the back of your head and continue to sense the feelings in your body.

BEING AND ENERGY

This exercise activates pressure points on the knee and foot. When you finish sit in the sitting posture for five to ten minutes, continuing to expand your feelings and sensations.

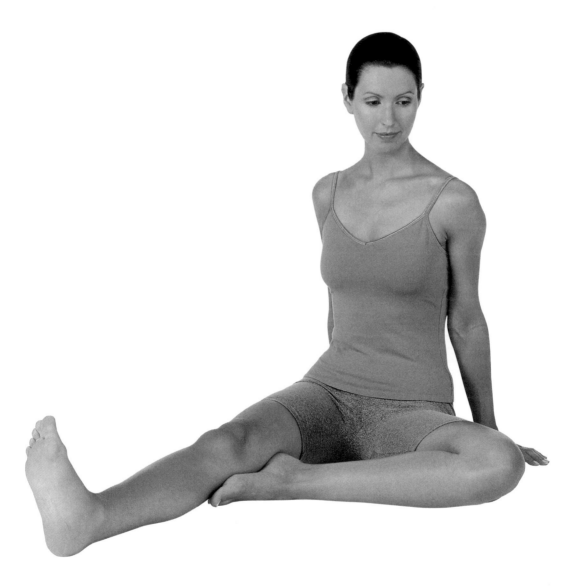

Sit on the floor with your palms on the floor near your hips and your right leg stretched out in front of you. Flex your right ankle so that the toes point upward and place your left foot against the inside of your right knee with your left knee on the floor. Push your left foot against your

right knee, and your right knee against your left foot until your legs are almost shaking. You may be able to push harder with the left leg than with the right. Hold the tension for 30 seconds to 1 minute, with your stomach relaxed, breathing easily through both nose and mouth.

Slowly release the tension, unifying breath, awareness and sensation and allowing the flavours of feeling to merge and expand. Rest here, expanding the sensations further. Then reverse the position of the legs and repeat the action. Do the entire exercise 3 times.

TRANSFORMING ENERGY

Through this exercise, mental agitation and emotional discomfort can be transformed. As soon as energy is disconnected from a particular pattern, new ways of being can form. Try this exercise when you feel tired, depressed, negative or blocked. The exercise can also be done sitting. At the end of the exercise, sit in the sitting posture for five to ten minutes, expanding the sensations stimulated by producing and releasing tension in this way.

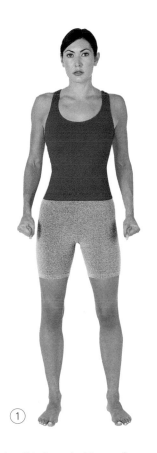

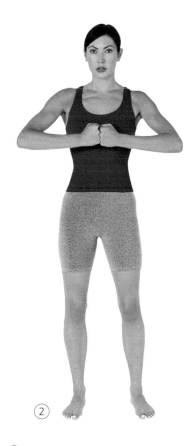

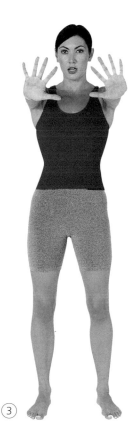

1 Stand well-balanced with your feet a comfortable distance apart, your back straight and your arms by your sides. Clench your fists strongly, hold your breath slightly and tighten your chest until you feel something similar in quality to anger.

2 Breathing very lightly – without losing the feeling of holding back in the chest – press your fists together, knuckle to knuckle, and place them in the centre of your chest. Make your body and fists very strong and tense. Inhale deeply so that your breath rolls down into your stomach and draws energy from the base of your spine up into your chest. Contain this energy internally, as if protecting yourself. Intensify the feeling of holding back as much as possible so that your energy becomes concentrated.

3 Keeping the rest of your body still, suddenly thrust your arms forward, palms away from you, releasing all the gathered energy and tension – physical, mental and emotional – in an explosion. As you do so, exhale sharply, shouting "ha!" from your chest. Pause for a moment with outstretched arms, fingers wide. What is the feeling that you experience?

Now slowly lower your arms to your sides and stand quietly for a few minutes. Do the entire exercise 3 times.

ACTIVATING HEALING ENERGY

This exercise helps us to contact and use the subtle energies of our bodies to heal ourselves on all levels. At the end sit in the sitting posture for five to ten minutes, continuing to expand the feelings activated by the exercise. Try a variation of this exercise with the knees bent: experiment to see how feeling is affected by different degrees of bending in the knees.

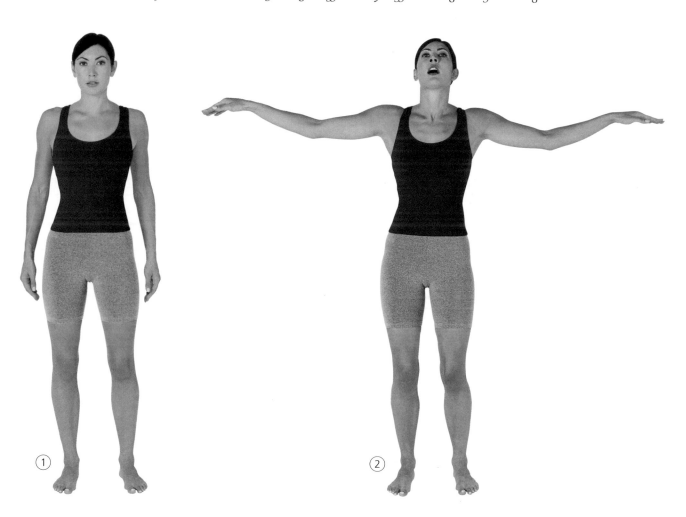

❶ Stand well-balanced with your feet about 6 inches (15cm) apart, your back straight and your arms relaxed at your sides.

Discontinue the exercise if you feel strong heat rising up your spine. Instead, gently lower your arms, straighten your head and sit in the sitting posture for 5 to 10 minutes, expanding the sensations in your body.

❷ Stretch your arms out to your sides at shoulder-height, palms down. Lift your head slightly to look at the point where the wall meets the ceiling. Relax your neck, open your mouth and flare your nostrils. Breathe softly and evenly through both nose and mouth. Relax your stomach and chest as fully as you can, tighten your buttocks and bring your attention to the base of your spine. If you feel something there, perhaps heat or a tingling

sensation, try to expand that feeling to the rest of your body. If mild shaking or trembling develops, explore the sensations and release the tension.

After holding the position for 3 to 5 minutes, slowly lower your arms to your sides, straighten your head and stand relaxed for several minutes, expanding the sensations in your body. Do the entire exercise 3 times.

CHANNELLING BODY ENERGY INTO THE SENSES

This exercise revitalizes the senses, sharpening sensory awareness. If you are an older person unused to regular exercise, it is best to avoid this exercise, which is a little strenuous. When you finish rest on your back for five to ten minutes, keeping your arms outstretched at shoulder-height, palms up, as you continue to amplify and extend the sensations in your body.

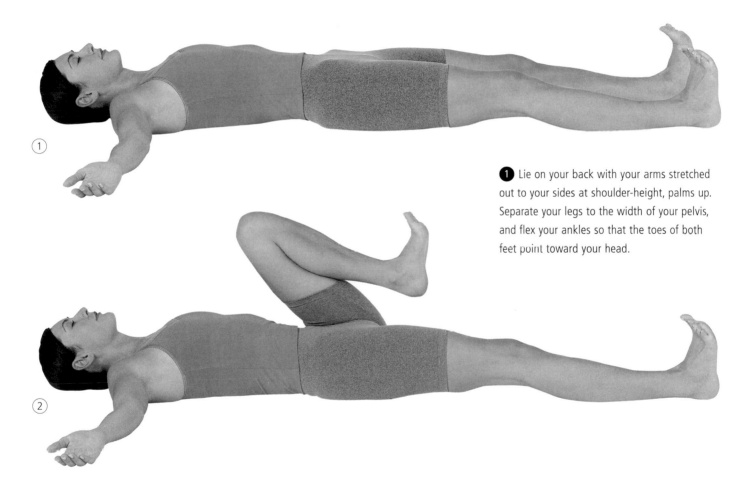

❶ Lie on your back with your arms stretched out to your sides at shoulder-height, palms up. Separate your legs to the width of your pelvis, and flex your ankles so that the toes of both feet point toward your head.

❷ Sliding your heel along the floor until it lifts naturally, bend your left knee and draw your thigh strongly toward your torso, while keeping your right leg straight. Breathing softly through both nose and mouth, hold the tension in your legs and feet for 15 to 30 seconds, keeping arms and shoulders relaxed.

Very slowly release the tension, straighten your leg and relax your feet, expanding the sensations stimulated by producing and releasing tension in this way. Rest briefly on your back before repeating the exercise on the other side. Do the complete exercise 3 times, resting for a few minutes after each repetition.

A variation of this exercise is done with both thighs pressed to the body at once; this version may produce more intense feelings.

WHOLENESS OF JOY

This exercise develops a sense of wholeness and connection. Do this exercise very gently if you are pregnant, have had any sort of back or neck injury, or have had an operation within the past three or four months. At the end rest in the sitting posture for five to ten minutes.

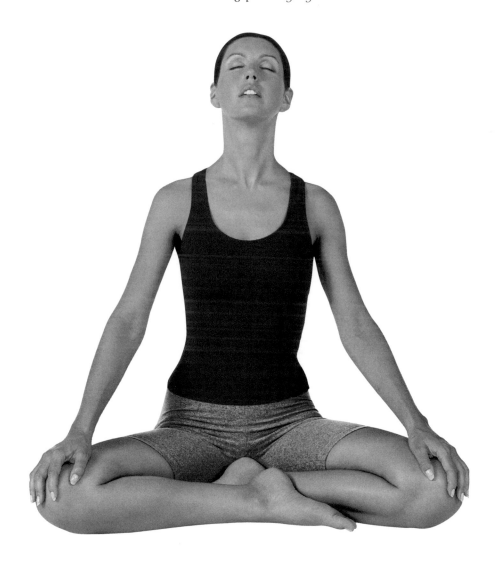

Sit cross-legged on a mat, cushion or low stool with your back straight. Grasp your knees firmly with your hands to create a feeling of strength in your arms, knees and hands, and lift your chest toward the ceiling. As your back arches, open your mouth and lift your chin. Do not let your head go all the way back – too extreme a curve in the neck will interrupt the flow of sensation. Breathe softly and evenly through nose and mouth. Relax your belly (this makes it possible to stretch the spine back a little more), taking care not to strain. Hold for 1 to 3 minutes, sensing the feelings in your chest and spine.

When you feel heat at the back of your neck, very slowly straighten your spine. As you release the tension, be aware of any sensations of heat and energy that extend beyond the ordinary limits of your body. Do the exercise 3 or 9 times, resting in the sitting posture for a few minutes after each repetition.

TOUCHING POSITIVE FEELING

This exercise stimulates joyful and loving feelings and activates sexual energies. At the end of the exercise, sit in the sitting posture for five to ten minutes, expanding and distributing the feelings awakened by the exercise.

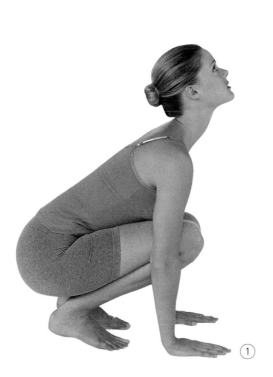

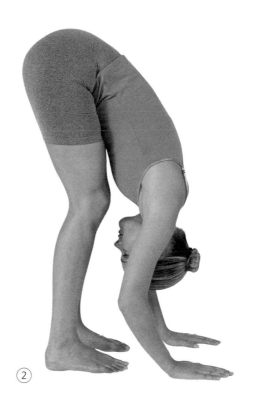

1 With your feet about 6 inches (15cm) apart, squat on the balls of your feet. With your arms outside of your legs, place your palms flat on the floor in front of you, fingers pointing forward. Look up toward the ceiling, breathing gently through nose and mouth.

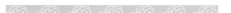

During the exercise you may feel warmth moving up your legs into your pelvis. Expand these sensations to your spine, upper body, arms and head. Feel them more. Allow them to permeate every cell in your body.

2 Keeping your palms flat on the floor, slowly lower your head, lift your pelvis toward the ceiling as far as possible without straining, and lower your heels to the floor. Feel the stretch in the backs of your legs. Hold for 30 seconds to 1 minute, relaxing your feet and stomach, letting your head hang loosely, and breathing as evenly as possible through both nose and mouth. If your legs tremble, explore the shaking and release tensions.

Slowly lower your pelvis, lift your head and heels, squat briefly on the balls of your feet, before sitting in the sitting posture for 1 to 2 minutes, expanding the sensations stimulated by the leg stretch. Do the exercise 3 times.

TEXTURE OF JOY

This exercise stimulates a sense of joy and encourages us to focus on and truly experience the full flavour of this feeling. At the end sit in the sitting posture for five to ten minutes, continuing to expand these sensations.

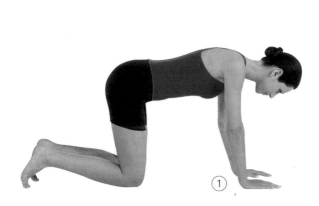

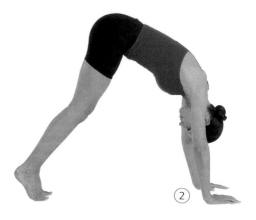

1 Get down on your hands and knees, (with a pillow beneath your knees if you prefer). Point your fingers forward. Lift your feet and put your toes on the floor so that your weight is balanced on your toes, knees and hands.

2 Keeping your palms flat on the floor and your arms straight, slowly lower your head, shift your weight forward a little and gently lift your knees until your legs are straight.

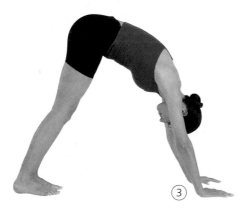

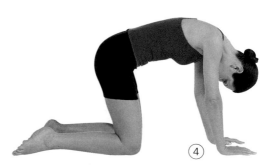

3 Lower your heels to the ground. Hold the stretch for between 30 seconds and 1 minute, breathing gently through both nose and mouth, and feeling the sensations in the backs of your legs. Let your head hang loosely from your neck. (If you cannot bring your heels all the

way to the ground, lower them as far as you can without straining the muscles in the backs of your legs, and hold the stretch in this position. Try bringing your hands closer to your body to decrease the stretch in the back of your calves.)

4 After 30 seconds to 1 minute, slowly lower your knees to the floor, sensing the feelings in your body as you release the stretch. Rest briefly on your hands and knees with your feet relaxed, soles up, continuing to expand your sensations. Perform the exercise 3 times.

HEART GOLD THREAD

This exercise balances the heart centre, increases mental and physical energy, builds strength and concentration, and improves the circulation and complexion. In addition the exercise can help to identify and transform psychological and physical blockages. At the end of the exercise, lie down on your back for ten minutes, continuing to amplify the sensations generated by the position until they spread beyond your body.

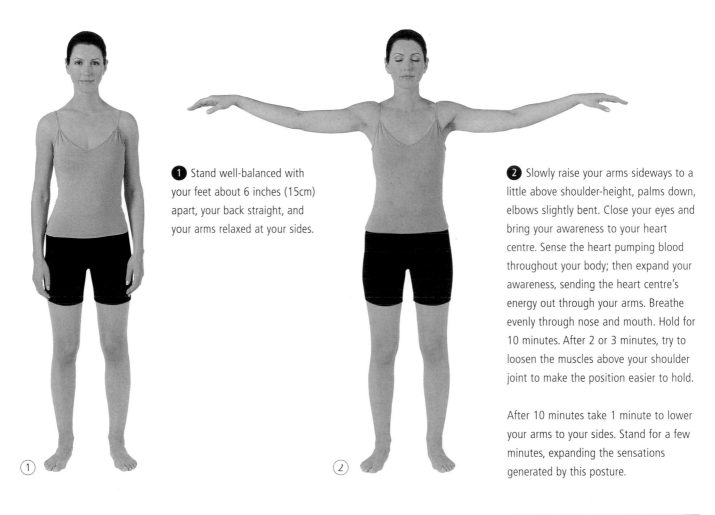

1 Stand well-balanced with your feet about 6 inches (15cm) apart, your back straight, and your arms relaxed at your sides.

2 Slowly raise your arms sideways to a little above shoulder-height, palms down, elbows slightly bent. Close your eyes and bring your awareness to your heart centre. Sense the heart pumping blood throughout your body; then expand your awareness, sending the heart centre's energy out through your arms. Breathe evenly through nose and mouth. Hold for 10 minutes. After 2 or 3 minutes, try to loosen the muscles above your shoulder joint to make the position easier to hold.

After 10 minutes take 1 minute to lower your arms to your sides. Stand for a few minutes, expanding the sensations generated by this posture.

While performing this exercise, the memory of an emotion may enter your mind, perhaps sorrow, hurt or pain. Expand the feeling as much as you can, letting your mind and senses become one. Stay with the feeling until you penetrate it, releasing it into pure experience. A flash of energy (the energy of that memory) then enters the present and the pattern of the emotion melts away. Practised regularly, this exercise brings a constant sense of union, a willingness to let feelings arise and expand. Then we can face pain, fear and tension directly, releasing them as they occur in daily life.

As you become more familiar with this exercise, you can try holding the position for longer periods of time, up to 25 minutes. After completing the exercise you should rest for as long as you held the position, either standing with your arms relaxed by your sides and then lying down, or, if you prefer, simply lying down.

EXPANDING INNER ENERGY

This enjoyable exercise encourages the free flow of pure energy throughout the body, promoting positive feelings of happiness. At the end of the exercise, rest on your back with your legs outstretched for five to ten minutes, expanding the sensations stimulated by this movement.

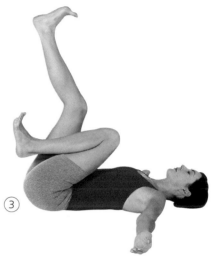

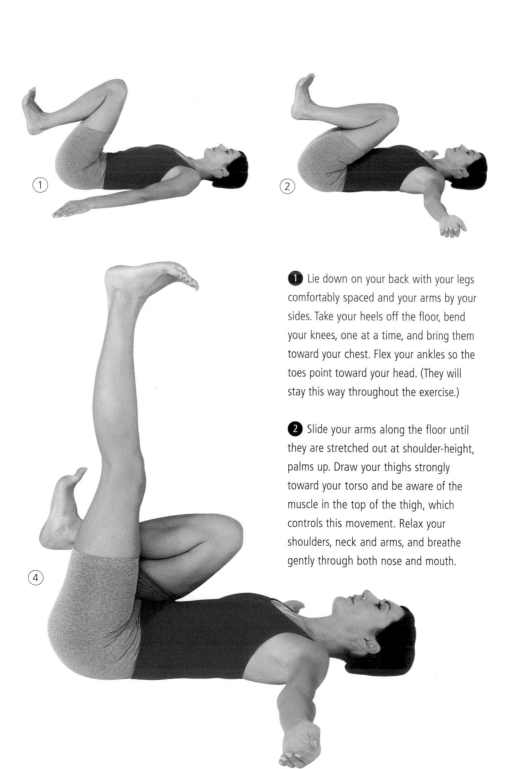

❶ Lie down on your back with your legs comfortably spaced and your arms by your sides. Take your heels off the floor, bend your knees, one at a time, and bring them toward your chest. Flex your ankles so the toes point toward your head. (They will stay this way throughout the exercise.)

❷ Slide your arms along the floor until they are stretched out at shoulder-height, palms up. Draw your thighs strongly toward your torso and be aware of the muscle in the top of the thigh, which controls this movement. Relax your shoulders, neck and arms, and breathe gently through both nose and mouth.

❸ Keeping your left thigh as close to your body as possible, slowly extend your right leg (with the ankle flexed) toward the ceiling. Feel the contraction in the left thigh and the extension in the right.

❹ Keeping your stomach and upper body relaxed, slowly bend the right knee, bringing the right thigh as close to your body as you can, while extending the left leg up. Let breath and awareness expand your sensations and become one with the movement.

Do the complete movement 3 times continuously. Then lower the left leg, release the tension and, one at a time, return your feet to the floor.

When you become familiar with the exercise opposite, try this variation.

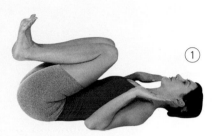

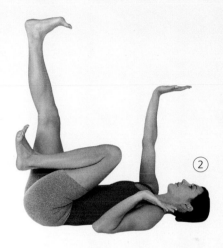

1 Lie on your back, legs a comfortable distance apart, arms close to your body, bent at the elbows so that the palms face the ceiling. Bend your knees, one at a time, bringing them close to your chest and flex your ankles. Imagine that a strong force is pushing against your hands, creating tension in your arms as well as in your legs.

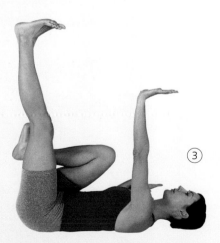

2 Maintaining the tension in your left arm and leg, slowly extend both your right arm (with the palm facing the ceiling) and your right leg (with the ankle flexed) toward the ceiling.

3 Then slowly bend and lower your right arm and leg, bringing them close to your body, and, at the same time, extend your left arm and leg.

Do the complete movement (including both sides of the body) 3 times continuously. Then slowly lower your left arm and leg, and release the tension in both arms and legs. Bring your feet back to the floor one at a time, straighten your legs, and bring your arms to your sides. Rest on your back for 5 to 10 minutes, breathing gently and evenly through both nose and mouth and expanding the sensations awakened by this movement.

ENERGIZING BODY AND MIND

This exercise relieves tension in the spine and lower back, thereby revitalizing the entire body and mind.
When practising this exercise you may feel heat between the shoulder blades
and sensations of opening in your lower energy centres.

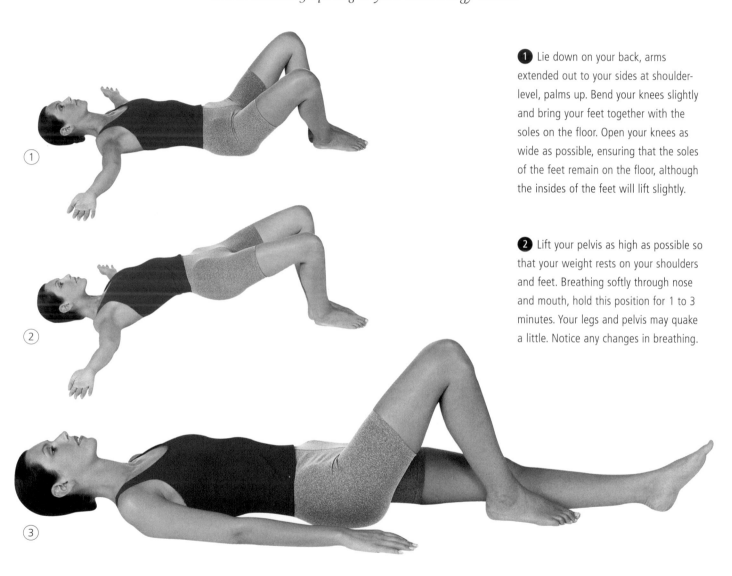

1 Lie down on your back, arms extended out to your sides at shoulder-level, palms up. Bend your knees slightly and bring your feet together with the soles on the floor. Open your knees as wide as possible, ensuring that the soles of the feet remain on the floor, although the insides of the feet will lift slightly.

2 Lift your pelvis as high as possible so that your weight rests on your shoulders and feet. Breathing softly through nose and mouth, hold this position for 1 to 3 minutes. Your legs and pelvis may quake a little. Notice any changes in breathing.

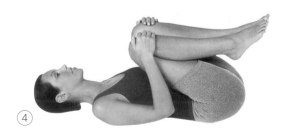

3 After 1 to 3 minutes, slowly lower your pelvis to the floor, straighten your legs one at a time, and bring your arms to your sides. Rest for a few minutes, expanding the feelings stimulated by this exercise. Do the exercise 3 times, resting after each repetition.

4 To finish, draw your knees toward your chest, place your hands on your knees and rest in this position for 5 to 10 minutes.

TRINITY OF PRACTICE: BREATH, ENERGY AND AWARENESS

This exercise stimulates and revitalizes inner energies, and builds strength and concentration. As you practise you may feel openings along your spine and in your chest, hands, neck and head. At the end sit in the sitting posture for fifteen minutes, broadening your sensations until they spread out to the universe and you are aware of nothing else.

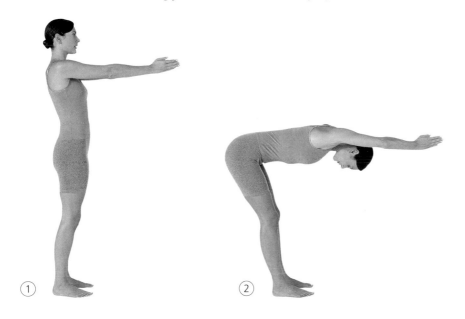

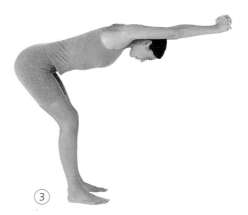

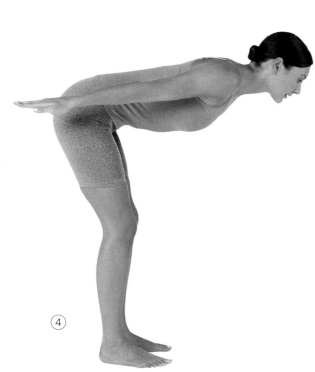

❶ Stand well-balanced, feet slightly apart, back straight, arms relaxed at your sides. Extend your arms in front, palms together, fingers pointing forward.

❷ In one continuous movement, stretch your arms forward and push your pelvis back, lowering your head between your arms until your torso, head and arms are parallel to the ground. Keep your back straight throughout this movement.

❸ In this position, stretch forward with the arms and backward with the pelvis, keeping your knees straight. Breathe as evenly as possible through both nose and mouth. Interlace the fingers and stretch further, in both directions (your body will

lower a little) until you feel you have touched a place of energy. You may begin to shake. Hold for 15 to 30 seconds.

❹ Without releasing the tension, slowly move your hands apart and keeping your arms at the same level, move them in an arc, palms down, until they are by your sides, pointing behind you. Stretch your neck forward and your pelvis back. Hold for as long as you can, breathing evenly through both nose and mouth.

Slowly release the tension and stand up. Stand silently for 3 to 5 minutes. Then repeat the exercise twice, resting after each repetition.

THE VALUE OF RETREAT

*"Everything you do can be a beautiful ceremony,
a dance of appreciation."*

Taking a brief retreat in a natural setting once, twice or even several times a year, can greatly expand your practice of Kum Nye. If possible you should spend four days each season or one week a year, either in the mountains, in a forest, or near an ocean or river.

During the retreat, try to spend as much time outside as you can. In the mornings, sit outside and practise breathing for about an hour. Adopt the sitting posture, gently open your mouth and nostrils, and breathe very, very slowly, holding your belly in slightly. Open all your senses and invite the living energies around you to enter your body. Allow your whole body, even your toes and your hair, to sense the energies of the cosmos – those of the light, the air, the earth, the plants, the water and the sky.

Visualize the positive healing qualities of these living energies as they flow into you and collect in your body. Mix your feelings with these energies before letting them radiate outward from you, linking you to the cosmos in an ongoing exercise, a continuing interaction, a circular dance of energy.

Continue this healing interaction of inner and outer energies while sunbathing twice a day for about twenty-five minutes (you should sunbathe for no longer than forty minutes at a time). After sunbathing or before sleeping, do an hour of massage, always rubbing oil into your body when you finish.

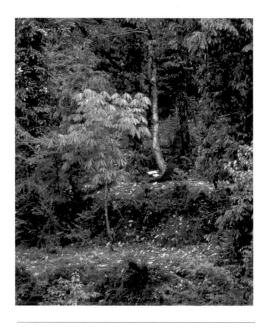

Inset: A Tibetan nun meditates in a forest. Time spent amid the vital energies of nature can restore to us a sense of wholeness and calm that is deeply relaxing. Kum Nye practised in natural settings is especially beneficial, as it attunes us to nature's healing power.
Opposite: This image shows the Himalayas near Gangotri in India. Vistas of earth and space, such as this, remind us that we are part of a larger reality, freeing our minds from preoccupations and allowing us to hear the primeval wisdom of our embodiment.

Massaging yourself outdoors using sesame oil is a particularly delicious experience that stimulates and opens all the senses. At some point during the day, practise one or two movement exercises that you wish to develop, bringing your awareness to the mantric syllables "Om Ah Hum" from time to time as you do so.

During the course of the retreat, and ideally throughout the rest of the year as well, you should sleep for seven or eight hours a night and eat simple, balanced meals. Whatever the nature of your diet, try to lighten it a little: avoid white flour, refined sugar and saturated fats, and eat more fruit, vegetables, nuts, seeds, soya products, pulses and wholegrains. Cut down on meat so that your diet becomes more than sixty-five per cent vegetarian. Always chew slowly and thoroughly, enjoying fully the various different tastes and textures of your food. To avoid bloating, try to finish eating when your stomach is half-full.

Throughout your daily activities, whether you are at home or on retreat, try to bring your body, mind and senses together by maintaining gentle, even breathing and adopting an attitude of relaxed, mindful concentration. When you live your life in this way, everything that you do becomes a beautiful act of ceremony; you will enjoy a permanent sense of wholeness, unity and fulfilment, an overwhelming joy that touches all aspects of your life as well as the lives of those around you.

THE NYINGMA INSTITUTE

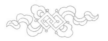

Based in Berkeley, California, the Nyingma Institute is a secular educational centre, a place where members of the public can investigate the teachings of the Tibetan Buddhist tradition and explore the applications of those teachings to Western lifestyles. The Institute, which was founded in 1972 by Tarthang Tulku (see p.9), offers a full range of classes, workshops and retreats in Kum Nye Relaxation, Nyingma Psychology, Meditation, Tibetan Language and Culture, and the essential principles of Buddhist teachings. An extensive program of Buddhist Studies covers the therapeutic applications of Buddhist teachings, and progresses to in-depth study of the *Sutras* (the Buddha's teachings), the *Abhidharma* (the study of mind and mental events) and the works of some of the great Buddhist philosophers. Residential programs include the four-month Human Development Training Retreat (see pages 9 and 137) and the two-month Integration Retreat. These retreats are designed to activate inner resources, revitalize the psyche and bring focus and balance to all aspects of life.

Most Institute workshops and retreats include the practices of Kum Nye Relaxation, which is a system of balancing and integrating the energies of body and mind based on the principles of the Tibetan medical system, and adapted specifically to meet Western needs. In the context of meditation, students are taught to use Kum Nye to calm the body and bring the mind to an alert yet gentle focus that leads naturally into meditation. In more content-oriented sessions, Kum Nye refreshes the student's body and awakens his or her mind, promoting an energized yet effortless concentration.

In 1977 Tarthang Tulku set down his most helpful Nyingma teachings in several books that were published in the Nyingma Psychology Series. He then worked with the faculty of the Nyingma Institute to create educational programs based on these books. By that time, Kum Nye Relaxation had already become an important course of study. Psychologists and health professionals, even those familiar with a wide range of therapeutic exercise and massage techniques, recognized Kum Nye's healing potential and urged Tarthang Tulku to publish details of his exercises. Great care was given to selecting and describing Kum Nye exercises that readers could do on their own, progressing from basic breathing and massage techniques to movement exercises appropriate for beginners as well as advanced practitioners. The result was *Kum Nye Relaxation* – the first presentation in book form of the system developed by Tarthang Tulku – produced by Dharma Publishing in 1978.

As well as producing the Nyingma Psychology Series, Dharma Publishing (founded by Tarthang Tulku in 1971) also supports the Nyingma Institute's educational programs by publishing translations of traditional Buddhist texts and introductions to Buddhist history, art and culture. Under its founder's guidance, Dharma Publishing has produced major collections of traditional Tibetan texts, including *The Nyingma Edition of the Tibetan Buddhist Canon* and *Great Treasures of Ancient Teachings*, a compilation of more than 80,000 texts in 639 atlas-sized volumes.

Since 1978 Tarthang Tulku has continued to direct the development of the Nyingma Institute's curriculum, designing programs and training its teachers and administrators. In particular, he introduced a rigorous teacher's training and certification program, with the result that authorized Kum Nye teachers could begin to offer seminars sponsored by study groups internationally. Kum Nye became more widely known in Europe and Brazil during the 1980s, when *Kum Nye Relaxation* was translated into German, Dutch, Italian and Brazilian Portuguese. In 1989 three Kum Nye study groups became branch Nyingma Institutes: one formed in Amsterdam, Holland; another in Münster, Germany (which has now moved to Köln); and a third was established in São Paulo, Brazil. A fourth institute formed in Rio de Janeiro, Brazil, in 1996. Today, all these institutes have authorized instructors with extensive experience of teaching Kum Nye and guiding individuals in the development of their own practice. Regular classes and workshops in Kum Nye Relaxation are offered at each institute throughout the year, and teachers from these institutes travel around the world to offer Kum Nye workshops throughout Europe and South America. (Please contact each centre directly for details of their full schedule.)

Two- and four-month residential programs incorporating Kum Nye are offered regularly at the Nyingma Institute in Berkeley. One-week and two-week Kum Nye residential retreats are regularly offered in the autumn, spring and summer, as well as around major holidays. The residential retreats and programs are specifically designed to accommodate people who come from distant areas or other countries. Other centres are also currently developing residential programs.

Today at the Berkeley Nyingma Institute, Kum Nye continues to play a large part in study courses and retreats, with the result that thousands of participants have experienced its benefits. The classes and workshops that focus specifically on Kum Nye usually consist of one-hour class sessions that incorporate breathing and massage techniques with a wide range of movement exercises and seated meditation practice. This gives participants opportunities to explore the potential in all these areas and create their own routine based on the exercises they find especially beneficial. Kum Nye residential retreats are held regularly throughout the year, allowing students to deepen their understanding through dedicated periods of intensive practice. Institute teachers may also introduce movement exercises in classes devoted to specific subjects, such as Buddhist psychology, philosophy and history. Kum Nye remains an important component of the Institute's annual Human Development Training Retreat, which incorporates physical movement, meditation and Tibetan insights into mind and mental development. A statement by Tarthang Tulku summarizes the point of this particular course: "Over time, pressure and tension demoralize and damage the human spirit. Loss of confidence, reluctance to take responsibility, and the feeling of being pressured, even controlled, are warning signs that our human spirit is being subjected to a dictatorship of some kind. But no matter where we look, it is difficult to find the root cause of pressured, anxious feelings. While we can point to certain events that seem to cause our tension, we forget to ask a more important question: why do we allow such things to control us? If we had the knowledge to direct our lives more skillfully, we could develop more inner freedom and confidence."

Practised regularly, Kum Nye allows the student to develop a deep sensitivity to the energies of body and mind and a fuller self-understanding based on the direct experience of emotions, thoughts, sensations and feelings. Beginners at the Nyingma Institute have found that the slow and gentle movements of Kum Nye offer a welcome experience of relaxation as stress melts away, sensory awareness is reawakened, the urgent chatter of thoughts is stilled, and mind and body become attuned. As students develop their practice of Kum Nye, they experience a marked reduction in stress levels together with a host of other benefits.

Intermediate students find that the restful discipline of familiar Kum Nye exercises is a reliable antidote to mental and emotional stress, a way to integrate the energies of body and mind and allow awareness to settle into a natural state in which insight arises as needed. As students learn to practise Kum Nye with patience and sensitivity, they can reliably select exercises to overcome specific physical problems, exercises that will counteract stiffness and rigidity while promoting muscle tone and circulation.

For advanced students, Kum Nye can work in concert with meditation practice to invigorate the body and invite deeper meditation experiences by loosening physical and mental rigidity. Often students have their first encounters with more fully grounded and alert states of mind while performing Kum Nye.

In this way, many students who come to the institute to practise Kum Nye with the intention of improving their general health and relieving stress have also discovered the benefits of meditation. Some have gone further to study the concepts that underlie both Kum Nye and meditation, and support a broader understanding of spiritual, emotional and mental health.

The following Nyingma Institutes are fully qualified to offer programs in Kum Nye Relaxation:

Nyingma Institute
1815 Highland Place
Berkeley CA 94704, USA
Tel: 001-510-843-6812
Fax: 001-510-486-1679
E-mail: Nyingma-Institute@nyingma.org
Website: www.nyingmainstitute.com

Nyingma Centrum Nederland (founded 1989)
Reguliersgracht 25, 1017 LJ
Amsterdam, The Netherlands
Tel: 0031-20-620-5207
Fax: 0031-20-622-7143
E-mail: nyingmacentrum@nyingma.nl
Website: www.nyingma.nl

Instituto Nyingma do Brasil (founded 1989)
Rua Cayowaa 2085 – Sumaré
01258-011 São Paulo, Brasil
Tel: 0055-11-3864-4785
Fax: 0055-11-3673-0292
E-mail: nyingmasp@nyingma.com.br
Website: www.nyingma.com.br

Nyingma Zentrum Deutschland (founded 1989)
Siebachstrasse 66
Köln, Germany
Tel: 0049-221-589-0474
E-mail: NyingmaD@aol.com

Centro Nyingma do Rio de Janeiro (founded 1996)
Rua Casuarina 297, Casa 2
Rio de Janeiro RJ
CEP 22260-160, Brasil
Tel: 0055-21-2527-9388
Fax: 0055-21-2579-1066
E-mail: nyingma@barralink.com.br

FURTHER READING

Nyingma Psychology Series

The following books are authored by Tarthang Tulku and published by Dharma Publishing (Berkeley, California). They present the core teachings of the Nyingma Institute:

Reflections of Mind

Gesture of Balance

Openness Mind

Kum Nye Relaxation, Parts 1 and 2

Skillful Means

Hidden Mind of Freedom

Knowledge of Freedom

Translations of Buddhist works (Dharma Publishing)

Works on meditation

Longchenpa *Kindly Bent to Ease Us, Parts I–III* (transl. Herbert V. Guenther), 1976. A guide to the Dzogchen path to enlightenment.

Mipham, Lama *Calm and Clear* (transl. with a commentary by Tarthang Tulku), 1973. Two practical guides to meditation by a leading nineteenth-century practitioner and scholar.

Biographies

Nam-mkha'i sNying-po *Mother of Knowledge: The Enlightenment of Ye-shes mTsho-rgyal* (transl. Tarthang Tulku and Jane Wilhelms), 1983. The story of Tibet's first female master.

Tsogyal, Yeshe *The Life and Liberation of Padmasambhava* (transl. Kenneth Douglas), 1978. A complete biography of Tibetan Buddhism's founder by his consort and principal disciple.

Voice of the Buddha (transl. Gwendolyn Bays). The Lalitavistara Sutra: the Buddha's own account of his birth, enlightenment and first teachings.

Introductions to Buddhism (Dharma Publishing)

Crystal Mirror Series (ed. Tarthang Tulku). Introductions to the historical and philosophical development of Buddhism in India, the Buddha and the masters who continued his teaching, and the transmission of Buddhism to Tibet.

Writings on Tibetan medicine (various publishers)

Clifford, Terry *Tibetan Buddhist Medicine and Psychiatry: The Diamond Healing*, Samuel Weiser (York Beach, Maine), 1990. (First published 1984.)

Donden, Yeshe and Hopkins, Jeffrey *Health Through Balance*, Snow Lion (New York), 1976.

Kunzang, Jampal (Ven. Rechung Rinpoche) *Tibetan Medicine Illustrated in Original Texts*, University of California Press (Berkeley and Los Angeles), 1976, and Wellcome Institute of the History of Medicine, the Wellcome Trust (London), 1973.

Khangkar, Lobsang Dolma *Lectures on Tibetan Medicine* (compiled and edited by K. Dhondup), Library of Tibetan Works and Archives (Dharamsala, India), 1986.

Fundamentals of Tibetan Medicine according to the rGyud-bzhi (transl. and ed. T. J. Tsarong et al), Tibetan Medical Centre (Dharamsala, India), 1981.

Mind and Mental Health in Tibetan Medicine, Potala Publications (New York), 1988. A collection of three essays previously published in *ReVision Magazine*, *Parabola Magazine* and *The Tibetan Review*: "Mind and Mental Disorders in Tibetan Medicine" by Mark Epstein and Sonam Topgay; "Sleep and the Inner Landscape", an interview with Dr. Yeshe Donden (transl. Robert Thurman); "Mind-Made Health: a Tibetan Perspective", adapted from a paper presented by Dr. Lobsang Rapgay at a medical conference in Australia, 1982.

Additional articles can be found in:

Tibetan Medicine: a publication for the study of Tibetan medicine, Library of Tibetan Works and Archives (Dharamsala).

INDEX

ACKNOWLEDGMENTS

Picture credits

The publisher would like to thank the following people, museums and photographic libraries for permission to reproduce their material. Every care has been taken to trace copyright holders. However, if we have omitted anyone we apologise and will, if informed, make corrections in any future edition.

Page 15 Ian Cumming, Tibet Images, London; **17** Ian Cumming, Tibet Images; **19** Ian Cumming, Tibet Images; **20** Diane Barker, Tibet Images; **134** Greta Jensen, Tibet Images; **135** Ian Cumming, Tibet Images

Publisher's acknowledgments

Duncan Baird Publishers would like to thank Elizabeth Cook, Margaret Mitchell, Ralph McFall, Joleen Vries and Charaka Jungens for all their hard work, support and dedication to this project.

Author's acknowledgments

Dharma Publishing would particularly like to thank Duncan Baird for his interest in Kum Nye, his willingness to work with us in the creation of this book, his generosity of heart, and his sincere motivation to publish books that have the potential to benefit others.

We would also like to thank all of the staff at DBP, who have worked with us so skillfully and patiently during the course of the project: Judy Barratt, for her enthusiasm and encouragement at the outset; Dan Sturges, for his tireless efforts to meet all of our requests; Nadia Mason for her cooperation and perseverance with the jackets; Matthew Ward, for his skilled figure photography; and Lucy Latchmore, for her fine editing of the text.